SPIRA SPEAKS
Dialogs and Essays on the Mucusless Diet Healing System
Volumes One, Two, and Three

By Professor Spira

What Others Are Saying about the Writings of Professor Spira

"I am amazed at your story. You really give hope to us all!"

-Kim Raylee (Ehret Club Member)

"First, I must say, thanks for the internet! It is a very nice, comforting feeling to be able to communicate with someone who has been successful with this diet, able to keep it simple, and answer questions. Thank you!"

-Tim Wader (Ehret Club Member)

"You truly are amazing. You have done nothing but given all you can to help me and I truly appreciate this. Thank you for feeding me."

-Samantha Claire (Pianist and Educator)

"I'm definitely impressed. As simple as you kept much of the language in the text, the writings resonate (with me) on a much deeper level. The reading forced me to reassess my personal perspective on the subject, and served to challenge all that I previously held to be true. I have much (more) work to do! Thanks again!"

-Danny Michael (Natural Health Consultant and Dietary Scientist)

"GREAT work! This actually answered a lot of my questions on various things. I think that it's a great source of material to reference for aspiring Ehretists everywhere. A lot of the stories and such are great accounts that people can learn from."

-Thomas Shaw (Mucusless Diet Practitioner and Raw-foods Advocate)

"A very good habit I have established for the past 4 years is the daily distilled water and lemon juice enemas (thanks to a suggestion of Spira and the "Cincinnati Guys"). These morning enemas help me to quickly free the last part of my intestine, feeling a great sensation of freedom and lightness at the highest levels that last all day long. It is a good habit like brushing my teeth! And it works great for me!"

-Aldo Bassi (Arnold Ehret Italia Member)

"I enjoyed reading your article, Prof. Spira. You cover some key points regarding cleansing the body. I'm currently rereading the *Mucusless Diet* and also just started reading *Rational Fasting*. Listening to your videos has intrigued my interest in Ehret's teachings. I've been doing a high-fruit diet for several years now, but see that I'm also eating some mucus-forming foods such as spelt and starchy veg's. I guess I'm in that slow transition mode and I do instinctively realize it's the best for me, as I have not been good to my temple for most of my life. I feel blessed to have come across this information at such a fairly young age and I thank you for your contribution."

-Angel (Raw foodist and practicing fruitarian)

"Your personal rediscovery of your radiant, intended self is amazing! Living examples, that's what people like you are, timeless individuals who live natural truth and telebeam it to others. . . .Your book really "speaks" to the amazing personal journey that you've undergone as well as your quest to influence others, educate, restructure the domain of jazz performance, and guide and lead other prospective Ehretists or those seeking greater health more generally. As long as I have known you, I have felt it crucial that you document your insights. The result is intimate, generous, and articulate. I enjoyed the balance of theory/research, poetry and conversation, and the power this kind of assortment has to appeal to different kinds of learners. It was really interesting to read through your coaching, guidance, motivations, and relationship-building processes throughout your conversations—really didactic and timely, illustrating the struggles that people face—economic, familial, opposition from society, personal, emotive, and coping strategies. I have to say also that reading through this really helped me to understand your perspectives a lot better and piece things together that were a little more scattered in my mind, beforehand. It's simply extraordinary and has influenced me in ways I didn't expect and has shaped my own health trajectory."

-Cy (Living-foods advocate and future nurse)

"Thank you for the excellent work! As someone who has struggled with the yo-yo approach to mucus-free foods, this was an eye-opening post. I appreciate it."

-Kenny William (Health Seeker)

"The people just finding out about the Mucusless Diet Healing System NEED this—people like me . . . even after years on a raw transition we need to know it's OK to transition any way that we can. If you knew how much suffering, physically and emotionally, not only from my own mind, but from the well-meaning raw foodists—you need to be pristine in your diet" one of the (popular people) told me as I was on my way to the ER with a pseudo-blockage. All I hear is raw—raw—raw—and I thought I was cured, and I was just getting started. Your book is already helping me in ways that I cannot express. I'm typing through tears. When I tried to eat cooked vegan before, the paralysis got worse—it was because it was not mucusless."

-Wendy Campbell (Detoxification Specialist and Raw-Foods Advocate)

SPIRA SPEAKS
Dialogs and Essays on the Mucusless Diet Healing System
Volumes One, Two, and Three

By Professor Spira

Rev. 5/1/2014

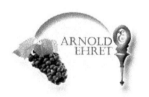

Breathair Publishing
Columbus, Ohio

Available from www.mucusfreelife.com, Amazon.com, Kindle, and other retail outlets

Printed in the United States of America

First Edition, 2013

Third Edition, 2014

ISBN-13: 978-0-99-065641-8
ISBN-10: 0-99-065641-1

www.mucusfreelife.com

Discover other titles by Breathair Publishing

Prof. Arnold Ehret's Mucusless Diet Healing System: Annotated, Edited, and Revised by Prof. Spira

Prof. Arnold Ehret's Rational Fasting for Physical, Mental and Spiritual Rejuvenation: Introduced and Edited by Prof. Spira

Thus Speaketh the Stomach and the Tragedy of Nutrition: Introduction by Prof. Spira

The Definite Cure of Chronic Constipation and Overcoming Constipation Naturally: Introduction by Prof. Spira

Coming Soon

Art of Transition: Spira's Mucusless Diet Healing System Menu and Recipe Guide

Robert Morse

The Great Lymphatic System

TABLE OF CONTENTS

i

Acknowledgments

I take little credit for the creation and content of these writings. It is a gift from the Universe. I am humbled and honored to have been given the privilege to channel and share the vibrations found within. A special debt of gratitude is due to Professor Arnold Ehret who authored the Mucusless Diet Healing System and Rational Fasting. Ehret rediscovered the key to unlock mankind's potential for superior health and spent his life healing the most terminal of patients. The following pages are but a profound testimony to the genius of his work. I also acknowledge the efforts of Ehret's chief associate Fred Hirsch, who played a major role in editing Ehret's written works and promulgating his message to the world.

A special recognition and debt of gratitude is due to my good friend and mentor Brother Air, who first introduced me to the works of Arnold Ehret. To date, Air has practiced the Mucusless Diet Healing System for over 30 years, and has elevated its practice as a lifestyle to incredible heights. Brother Air is certainly the most hardcore individual I know, yet he is also one of the most loving. He gives so much of himself to others and is constantly ready to help those in need. He is a true life artist and pioneer in the highest levels of health and vitality.

A special recognition and debt of gratitude is due to a modern-day sage and pioneer of Ehret's work, Victor Buttrom. It was Buttrom who first introduced the Mucusless Diet Healing System to Brother Air and founded a musical group in honor of Ehret's work called The Healing System. His knowledge and understanding of the Universe through the perspective of Ehret's vital principles was astounding. I spent many hours engaged in Socratic dialogs with this true philosopher, and much of my writings are directly inspired by his brilliance.

A special recognition is due to my brothers Daktehu, Baby Babaji, and "Uncle" Eddie Brookshire, whose music, love, and wisdom inspire me to achieve my full potential in all areas of my life. As musical brethren, there is nothing I enjoy more than making music with these giants in the Breathairean Ensemble.

I acknowledge the following individuals for their love, support, and inspiration over the years. Special thanks to my good friend Scott Martin (Raw Ehretist and owner of Eye-dye), whom I first met through the Online Ehret Club. As our web designer, he has been instrumental in allowing me and my colleagues to share our music and message with the world. Special thanks to Alvin Last, who became the custodian of Ehret Publishing following Fred Hirsch. As a result of his dedication, Ehret's primary works have remained in print and reasonably priced so that all may benefit. I also give special thanks to Luciano Gianazza, who has been the leading proponent of Ehret's teachings in Europe. Based in Italy, he has personally translated Ehret's works and has fostered a strong online community on his series of websites, including arnoldehret.it.

I would like to thank all whose conversations, questions, support, and interest in health have inspired me to share my perspectives and experiences through writing and music. Special thanks go to Ryan Wells, Loving Star, Tekoa, Benita, Khaleeq, Mawusi, the Children of the Sun, Angela, Ethel, Cy, Samantha, the Wader Family, Lorens Novosel, Dr. Washington, Jay, Rane Roatta, Bob, Deborah, Janaan Al Jahanni, the faithful listeners of our Immortality Pipeline radio show, Dan "the Life Regenerator" McDonald, Dr. Robert Morse, Wendy Dennis-Campbell, Thomas Shaw, Danny Michael, Victoria Bard, my Aunt Alice L. Noonan, my family, and the dedicated fans of the Breathairean Ensemble. And you, gentle reader, have my deepest gratitude for your interest in the highest levels of health, vitality, and physiological liberation.

Peace, Love, and Breath!

-Prof. Spira (December 2012)

Dedication

To Arnold Ehret, Fred Hirsch, and Vic

Preface

The following is a compilation of writings and dialogs that I exchanged with friends and family about my experiences practicing Prof. Arnold Ehret's *Mucusless Diet Healing System* over the past 10 years. When I first read the *Mucusless Diet*, I knew that I had obtained a document containing sacred and vital information about the true nature of the health of humankind. As a child, I watched my mother suffer and ultimately die of horrific health conditions. After spending countless hours in hospital rooms and nursing homes, I prayed that I might one day learn why humans must suffer such deplorable conditions. This prayer was answered after meeting Brother Air, who not only introduced me to the works of Prof. Arnold Ehret, but stood as a living example of how Ehret's work could be translated into a sustainable lifestyle. I was then introduced to a community of mucusless diet practitioners who created the support system that I needed to take on the challenging journey ahead of me. I must first express my appreciation to Brother Air and every member of the community for all their love and support over the past 10 years.

Within the first 6 months of practicing the diet, I lost 110 pounds and healed many of my ailments, including allergies, sleep apnea, daily migraine headaches, lower back pain, frequent indigestion, and yearly bouts of bronchitis. I quit taking the pharmaceutical medicines that I had endured since infancy and quelled all desires for meat, dairy, alcohol, tobacco, marijuana, and other questionable substances. In light of these remarkable results, I wanted to tell the world this great news: "It was rediscovered that the foundation of human illness is pus- and mucus-forming foods! Humans are a frugivorous species! The pain and suffering of humankind can be relinquished after being cleansed and rebuilt on the foods designed for humans!" Yet, I learned that most of my closest friends and family were not ready to encounter such information. I realized that this valuable knowledge was meant for me, and that I needed to run with it and transform myself before my desire to help others could be realized.

In 2003, I watched Brother Air sustain an 8½-month juice fast. After another year of intensive transition and study, I did my first extended juice fast of 6 months. At this point, I felt the need to document my journey. After a meeting with jazz saxophone legend Charles Lloyd, Brother Air and I were inspired to create the Breathairean Ensemble. It is a vegetarian jazz organization which includes mucusless diet practitioners. My primary vehicle for expressing this vital information became my music-making with the Breathairean Ensemble. We also started a radio show called the Immortality Pipeline on the local community radio station where we shared our music and experiences practicing the mucusless diet. As I began to promote the band on the internet, I realized that I was subsequently exposing people to, and educating people about, the *Mucusless Diet Healing System*. I began to seek out others interested in Ehret's work and found my way to the online Ehret Club Forum administered by Alvin Last. It was on this forum that I first wrote about the *Mucusless Diet*. As I spoke of my experiences and the thriving Ehretist community in Cincinnati, I began to receive many health-related questions. As I began to respond, I realized that these dialogs would be of great interest and importance to future generations of health seekers. In the years that followed, I interacted with many others interested in Ehret through YouTube, Facebook, the Ehret Italia Forum, and email.

I knew that the day would come when I would compile my writings and make them more available to the public. The following version contains much of the raw, mostly unedited, encounters that I have had with people about my experiences with the diet. As a consequence, the writings document my journey and those of others becoming mucusless. Some of the questions have been edited and names changed to protect the privacy of those with whom I am communicating. Today, the short eBook pamphlet is in fashion, and my writings have been organized into three volumes that cover different areas of interest and experience. In addition to short essays, dialogs comprise several chapters, many of a Socratic nature, which took place primarily in online forums or through private emails. In addition to learning practical information about transitioning to a mucus-free lifestyle, this eBook is designed to help you shift your consciousness toward a more natural dietetic paradigm free from modern medical errors and faulty assumptions. I highly recommend that you read Arnold Ehret's *Mucusless Diet Healing System* and *Rational Fasting* prior to, along with, or after this eBook. Although it is certainly not required, knowledge of Ehret's works will help you to fully benefit from this work.

Much has changed over the past 5 years as numerous self-identified raw foodists, fruitarians, and fasters use social-media sites to document and share their stories with others. There has been a major shift in the public consciousness as more people begin to seek out the truth about higher levels of health. Modern-day advocates for plant-based lifestyles have helped raise public awareness levels to a point where the information that we have may be more easily understood, respected, and practiced. Although we have only scratched the surface of humankind's potential to regain superior health, our experiences and information about sustaining a mucus-free lifestyle are vital to all who seek true wellness. Arnold Ehret is the forefather of modern plant-based, vegan, raw-foods living and mucus-free natural healing. Yet, too few people know of his works or the communities of people who currently live a mucus-free lifestyle. The world needs to be exposed to the power of the *Mucusless Diet Healing System* now more than ever!

With the support of my friends, family, and community, I am ready to tell the world our profound story . . .

VOLUME ONE (Fundamentals)

Chapter 1—Introductory Essays about Sustaining a Mucusless Lifestyle

A Profound Transition: Testimony of Prof. Spira Part 1

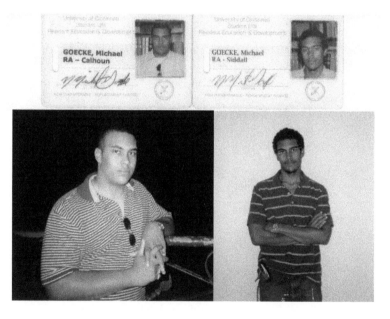

Top Left: Resident advisor ID taken September 2002 (280 lbs); Top Right: taken September 2003 (170 lbs). The bottom left photo was taken during a Boy Scout trip at Niagara Falls 2 years before starting the mucusless diet, and the bottom right is photo was posted on the "Meet your R.A.s" bulletin board in Siddall Hall at the University of Cincinnati.

I was addicted to pus- and mucus-forming foods. A lot of them. Well, I'm still an addict, but back then, a normal meal could consist of two chili-cheese footlong coneys, five root beers, popcorn, and a cheeseburger at our neighborhood Root Beer Stand.[1] Unfortunately, I was in a social setting and cultural landscape that gave me status for my big stature and indulgent lifestyle. I played American football and was a 250-pound varsity offensive lineman for the Princeton Vikings.[2] I loved the feeling of running onto the field while the crowd exploded with sounds of drunken joy, then legally running people over during the game. My other love was music. I had played the trombone since fifth grade and was fascinated with jazz. When it was time for college, I decided that I wanted to pursue my spiritual love of music and went to the University of Cincinnati College-Conservatory of Music[3] to study jazz.

When I began school, I thought I was on the right track. I was an "A" student in one of the top music schools in the country, experiencing the legal and illegal fun of American college life, while eating and drinking as much as I could take in. But this excessive lifestyle came with a cost, and I suffered from many ailments. I had chronic migraine headaches, joint pain, bad allergies, frequent nose bleeds, painful hemorrhoids, and yearly bouts of bronchitis.

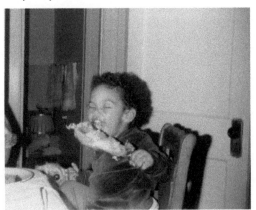

"Bam-Bam" Goecke with Turkey Leg, about age 4

1. For more information on the Sharonville, Ohio Root Beer Stand see: www.roadfood.com/Restaurant/Reviews/512/the-root-beer-stand.

2. To view the Iron Viking Creed see http://bit.ly/iron-viking-creed.

3. For more information about CCM see http://ccm.uc.edu/about.

As a child, I had tubes put in my ears to help drain large amounts of mucus from my sinuses and was injected with countless drugs. Around age 7, I began taking daily allergy medications. I first took Seldane, but after several years it was driven off the market for killing people. I then was put on Allegra, followed by Allegra D, then Zyrtec, Claritin (did nothing for me—like taking a sugar pill), and finally back to Allegra D. Along the way, I frequently took antibiotics, migraine medicine, and many over-the-counter drugs. In junior high and high school, I had doctor's orders that allowed the school nurse to supply me with Advil. I had splitting headaches almost every day and often left class to take an Advil and lie down in the nurse's office. In addition, my nose was often red, sore, and scabbed from blowing it hundreds of times a day . . . almost every day.

By the time I went off to college, I weighed over 280 pounds. I planned to move into the dorms, but I was self-conscious about my loud snoring. My Boy Scoutmaster had used a CPAP unit[4] and he said it cured his snoring. I went to the doctor for a sleep study and was hooked up to dozens of wires, given a lot of junk-food snacks to eat, and told to fall asleep. Needless to say, I did not get much rest. The doctor promptly diagnosed me with sleep apnea[5] and ordered me to purchase a CPAP unit. Thus, I was 19 years old and already hooked up to a respirator at night.

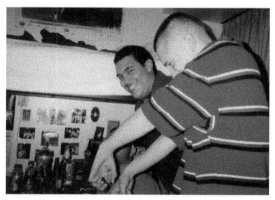

280 pounds, drunk in college dorm c. 2002

---

4. For information about the continuous positive airway pressure machine (CPAP), see http://en.wikipedia.org/wiki/C-PAP.

5. Sleep apnea is a type of sleep disorder characterized by pauses in breathing or instances of shallow or infrequent breathing during sleep.

3

I felt as if I had no control over my health and I would joke with friends that I would probably have my first stroke by age 26. Up to this point, I had been exposed to many of the popular dietary fads and had investigated a few of them without being impressed or successful. I worked out constantly, took diet pills, ginger root supplements, and more in futile attempts at losing weight. I watched every late-night infomercial on diet and exercise, fantasizing about the possibility of actually gaining control over my weight. Yet, I was not really interested in true health but only in looking fit and being buff. Unfortunately, none of the diets being pushed in the mainstream made any sense to me. So I decided to just over-indulge in food with the philosophy that I would just "die whenever it was time for me to go." But, when I left high school, I stopped working out like a varsity athlete. Instead, I practiced my trombone for 8 to 12 hours a day. I ate huge meals and then practiced for hours, taking breaks only to smoke and eat candy bars or Doritos.

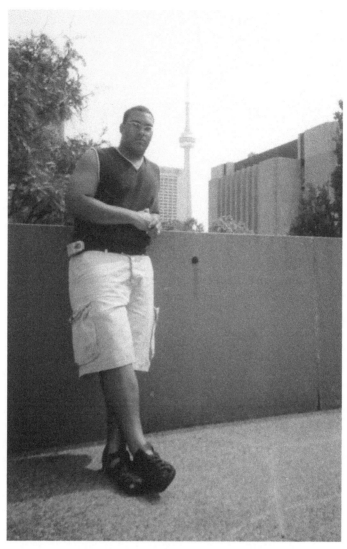

250 pounds, c. 2000 in Toronto, Canada

During my freshman year, I made it a point to plug into the local jazz scene to supplement my school activities. I knew that I would really learn how to play music while on the professional jazz bandstand, and I sought out as many opportunities as I could. On Sunday nights, I would go to Sonny's jazz jam session and sit in with my trombone. Sonny's was one of those bars where the older black folks congregated to drink and socialize. The older men would show off their *brand new* 1967 leisure suits, while the older women would get wasted and try to offer me drinks saying, "You so fine, baby!" And of course, the old sugar daddies would show up courting their young sugar babies. One Sunday I met an interesting jazz drummer named Brother Air.[6] After seeing him around Cincinnati at other local jazz spots, I began to talk with him about health and diet. Air dismissed the principles of Western dietetic theory and asserted that the only true road to health was through Prof. Arnold Ehret's *Mucusless Diet Healing System*. Brother Air said that he was over 40 years old and had practiced the diet for more than 20 years. This was shocking, as he did not look anywhere near 40 years old.

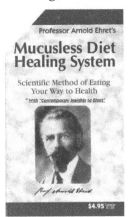

One evening, my saxophonist friend Daktehu[7] and Brother Air were sitting in on Erwin Stuckey's set at Chez Nora in Northern Kentucky. At the intermission, Daktehu and I hit the free buffet and filled our plates with chicken wings and other delectable items. As we sat and ate, Air began to speak very clearly about the *Mucusless Diet Healing System*. As the conversation progressed, Daktehu and I ate slower and eventually quit. As I looked at my plate with new eyes, Brother Air talked about his experience eating nothing but fruit for an entire year, and sustaining 100-day juice fasts. This caused something to click in my brain. Humans as fruit eaters! It made so much sense. If any being on the planet could subsist on nothing but fruit, why is it not possible for humans? By the end of the conversation, we had both decided to buy the *Mucusless Diet Healing System* and check it out.

6. For more information about Brother Air see www.mucusfreelife.com/popular/brother-air/

7. For more information about Daktehu see www.breathairmusic.com/band/bios/daktehu/.

After reading Arnold Ehret's *Mucusless Diet Healing System* and *Rational Fasting for Physical, Mental and Spiritual Rejuvenation,* my entire concept of life was transformed. The information seemed so simple, yet it challenged every assumption that I had about sickness and how the human body functions. For days, I sat and let questions flow through my mind: "Could this information really lead to the fountain of youth?" "Is the fundamental cause for aging and death mucus and pus?" "Is disease and sickness a self-induced thing?" "Did Brother Air really survive on nothing but fruit for an entire year?" "Are the lungs really the pump and the heart, the valve?" "If man is supposed to eat fruit, why did we start eating dead animals and cooked/fermented foods?" "Is eating protein-rich food really unnecessary and harmful?" "And what is so important about the fifth chapter of the *Mucusless Diet*?" "What is meant by the body being an "air-gas engine," and why was I instructed to read and reread this chapter about five times?" "What is meant by 'Vitality = Power – Obstruction'?"

One cool autumn day, I sat alone in a Memorial Hall practice room holding my silver trombone. I was dressed in a pair of brown suede, oxford pants and a yellow short-sleeved, 100 percent silk, button-up shirt—all from Bachrach Men's Clothier where I had been a sales representative. I sighed. On the wall stood a big mirror with a pattern of cracks in the bottom right hand corner, possibly left by the angry hand of some hopeless music student before their board examination. I gazed at 280 pounds of swollen anguish wrapped in fine fabrics. At that moment, my life blazed before my eyes. I thought about the instances when I had been ridiculed for being fat. I remembered the indescribable pain of seeing my grandmother and mother pass away due to chronic illnesses. I tried to imagine how many thousands of tissues had rubbed my sore, scabbed nose over the years. I remembered how unfulfilled I felt when I smoked or drank. I thought about the overall suffering of humanity. Is eating solely to blame for the ills of humankind? This was followed by a vision of the future. A future when all people would be empowered to seek superior health through a lifestyle that is in tune with Nature's laws. An era when concepts of pain, suffering, and death are remembered only through ancient tales and legends. It was at that moment that I became filled with the unrelenting determination to do all in my power to transform myself through this profound information that I had the privilege to receive. I realized my opportunity was a rare and precious gift that very few people were given. I had information that held the potential to transform the entire Universe! I then wiped a tear

7

from my right eye and vowed to dedicate my life to pursuing superior health through the practice of the *Mucusless Diet Healing System.*

To be continued. . . .

Peace, Love, and Breath!

-Prof. Spira

What Do We Need To Eat? An Introduction to the *Mucusless Diet Healing System*

c. 2007

To eat or not to eat? That is indeed the question. Moreover, why do we eat? Do we eat to live or do we live to eat? Is there an answer to this great dietetic paradox that we must consume nutritious foods to live, but these foods may be the root cause of sickness and death? To investigate this paradox, we must ask: What does the body need? We know that people do not need dead animal flesh or frozen and fermented animal milk to live, yet people around the world consume them with impunity. We also know that rice can be cooked into sticky glue, yet it is a staple meal for many. We hear about people who can abstain from food for a short time, but how is this possible? If the body does not need dead animals or milky-gluey substances to survive, then what do we need? Given the above, it seems that the most important substance that we consume is air. People can do without meat, grain, starches, and carbs, but they cannot live without air. Thus, air is premium in our realities; but for many, it is the thing thought about the least.

I began to explore the needs of the human body about 8 years ago. I was in college studying jazz trombone performance in Cincinnati when I met a jazz drummer by the name of Brother Air performing at local jazz venues. Brother Air told me about the *Mucusless Diet Healing System* by Prof. Arnold Ehret, which he and his family had been practicing for the past 25 years. I was initially impressed by his stories of sustaining an all-fruit diet for a year and his concept of pus- and mucus-forming foods being the root cause of human illness. At the time, I was in bad shape. I weighed over 280 pounds and suffered from a variety of ailments, including: chronic migraine headaches, lower back pain, joint pain in my right hand from football, joint pain in my right knee, chronic allergies, and otolaryngological problems including chronic cases of bronchitis. At the age of 18, I began using a CPAP unit (a machine that pumps oxygen into the nose during sleep), and I was also an 11-year veteran of consuming daily doses of allergy medications. What was the cause of my illnesses? The doctors told me that it was probably genetic and that chronic illness runs in my family. According to doctors, it wasn't my fault; and the best way to battle my illnesses was finding the right drugs. Since I grew up with family members who took as many as 10 pills a day, organized in little plastic containers labeled M for Monday, T for Tuesday, etc., I equated adulthood with the amount of medications I took. Thus, sickness meant status and maturity. While growing up, I would brag to my friends about how I was already taking medicine like adults. An MRI at the age of 17 to investigate my unbearable migraine headaches felt like a rite of passage to me.

What the doctors did not consider telling me was that I needed to examine my dietary habits. They forgot to mention that it is not okay to eat a large double-pepperoni, bacon, and ham pizza without sharing it with friends. Or that eating two footlong cheese coneys and a cheeseburger in one sitting may be bad for my health. Or that it was unhealthy to eat a sack of 10 cheeseburgers, cheese sticks, and a chocolate malt from United Dairy Farmers all in one sitting. I learned that my pain and suffering could not be blamed on my family's genes or on God, as some people suggested, but that the food which I consumed was to blame for my sick and pathological condition. More specifically, mucus- and pus-forming foods were the problem.

In the *Mucusless Diet Healing System*, I was exposed to Arnold Ehret's Mucus Theory, which posits that mucus- and pus-forming foods (i.e., dead animal products, dairy, grains, and starches) are the fundamental cause of human illness. These are foods that have no nutritious value and cause the body's systems to become constipated over time. As we become more and more encumbered, our body reacts either by attempting to eliminate mucus (e.g., the so-called common cold) or by suppressing the immediate elimination, from which chronic illness and latent diseases will eventually emerge.

The mucus idea made sense, but it seemed too simple. I had been conditioned to believe that if I did not see a bunch of complicated medical terminology, then it could not be good physiological science. If pus and mucus could explain human illness, then why are there so many names for different diseases and ailments? I knew that I would need to test the Mucus Theory on my own body if I wanted to find out if it were true. At the time, I was living in a college dorm as a resident advisor. I was a sophomore and had endured my freshman year of unrestrained eating, drinking, and smoking a variety of substances. In fact, I had gained about 30 pounds during my freshman year of college. In addition to pizza, cheeseburgers, and fish sticks, the dorm cafeteria had many fruits and a great salad bar. I began to eat as much fruit and salad as I could and traded horrific mucus formers, such as cheeseburgers and eggs, for lighter mucuses, such as 100-percent-wheat spaghetti and tomato sauce. By trying to abstain from mucus, I quickly learned how addictive and stimulating it is. I would have mucus-withdrawal symptoms comparable to what heroin addicts describe when they are kicking their habit. Some people would blame my withdrawal symptoms on a lack of nutrients or protein; this is why many people are scared to follow through with such a dietetic endeavor. There were days when I endured great weakness and felt terrible. Was the weakness from the fruit I was eating? I learned that my weakness was not from mucus-free fruits, which are the most perfect human foods, but was a result of my body loosening and attempting to throw off the pools of dross that I had been accumulating since childhood. I decided to keep going forward and after a while, I gained in strength and vitality. I watched quarts of mucus drain from my body and, since I was not consuming as many mucus-forming substances, I began to heal. As my body grew progressively cleaner, it became easier to eat living foods and engage in fruit-juice fasts. Within 6 months, I had lost 100 pounds and was emancipated from the many ailments and medications that had enslaved me since childhood.

What Is the Mucusless Diet Healing System?

Physiological Liberation begins and ends with Prof. Arnold Ehret's *Mucusless Diet Healing System*. It contains the most profound rediscovery of the nineteenth and twentieth centuries: that the human body is an "air-gas engine"! It explains how every sick person has a mucus-clogged system, and that this mucus comes from undigested, uneliminated, unnatural food substances that have accumulated since childhood. It has proven to be the most successful "compensation action" and so-called "cure" against every type of disease and illness known to humans. By its systematic application, hundreds of thousands of patients declared incurable by the "medical authorities" could be healed.

The *Mucusless Diet* consists of all kinds of raw and cooked fruits, starchless vegetables, and cooked or raw, mostly green-leaf vegetables. The *Mucusless Diet Healing System* is a combination of individually advised long- and short-term fasts, menus that progressively change to non-mucus-forming raw foods, and regular colon irrigation. In the book, Ehret observes that the human body is an air-gas engine that is maintained solely through breathing and that the accumulation of uneliminated waste materials (i.e., pus, mucus, and white dead blood) is what leads the chronically ill body to its painful demise. Ehret offers the equation, Vitality = Power - Obstruction, as an eloquent solution to the most injurious dietetic and physiological paradox in history: the belief

11

that our body needs to consume *nutritious* materials that will ultimately promote its death. He criticizes many of the commonly held theories of metabolism, protein, and nutrition, and offers new physiological explanations derived from experimenting with his Mucus Theory. Ehret's findings suggest that our bodies do not need to take in illness-causing substances to live, and that pus- and mucus-forming foods are the greatest proponents of human illness. Thus, the most fundamental human right is that we do not need to consume harmful, mucus-forming foods. In other words, we need not consume that which is unnecessary and damaging to human life.

Peace, Love, and Breath!

-Prof. Spira

General Information about the Mucusless Diet Healing System

Food Categories

Mucus-Forming Foods:

Meat, Poultry, Dairy, Grains, & Starches.

Meat, poultry, and dairy are the most dangerous mucus formers and should be avoided from the beginning. I used certain grains and starches, such as well-toasted 100 percent sprouted-wheat bread and 100-percent-wheat spaghetti as early transitional mucuses, that is, mucus-lean options.

Mucusless Foods:

Starchless/Fatless Fruits and Green, Leafy Vegetables

Deceptive Mucus Formers:

Here is a list of foods that many people do not realize create mucus:

Rice (great for creating glue to bind books, bad for the transition)

Avocados (fatty item that may be used on the transition, but are highly addictive. Although technically a fruit, if used, it is best to combine them with a combination salad or vegetables to aid elimination. However, it is recommended to stay away from them if you are not already stuck to them.)

Nuts (mucus-forming, but may be used on the transition; they are best eaten them with dried fruits like raisins to aid elimination)

Plantains (starchy)

Tofu (slimy and mucus-forming)

Unripened fruits like green bananas (the riper the fruit you eat, the better)

Corn (does not eliminate well; when cooked, it becomes mushy in the intestines)

Corn chips (Some people use them on the transition; but they are very addictive and do not eliminate well)

Beans (starchy and mucus-forming, but, they may be used sparingly on the transition within close proximity to green, leafy salads)

13

Good Transitional Habits to Remember

Avoid drinking with meals. If you must drink after a meal, wait at least 5 minutes before doing so. Wait more than 30 minutes if possible. Mixing liquid with solid food impedes the body's ability to digest and eliminate waste. The body craves simplicity and will eliminate better without such mixtures.

Most fruits and vegetables do not combine well. If you are eating a meal with fruits and vegetables, eat the fruits first—wait a few minutes, and then eat the salad/vegetables.

Eat no more than two meals a day, eliminating breakfast. Aim for an all-fruit meal in the afternoon and a combination salad/cooked vegetable meal in the evening. Fresh fruit and/or vegetable juices may be consumed throughout the day.

Always combine mucus-formers with salad and vegetables. On days when old mucuses are craved, use a transitional mucus and be sure to include a lot of salad and vegetables.

Do not be hard on yourself for craving mucus and eating some. Everyone falls off of the wagon sometimes, especially in the beginning. The key is to change your body's chemistry so that you no longer crave, or are even able to eat, the foods that are harmful to you. Mucus becomes about as appetizing as Clorox bleach.

Irrigate the colon with a (lemon) enema regularly.[8]

Surround yourself with supportive people. Misery loves company and eating is the greatest form of social unity known to humankind. Fruits and vegetables seem natural, but people conditioned and poisoned by Western dietary ideals often react with resentment and fear. Plug into positive people who are also interested in healing themselves.

Always follow a fast with a period of mucus-free menus. Do not break a fast with mucus-forming foods and be aware if you feel like you want to binge. If you have transitioned properly and have broken the fast effectively, you can avoid such problems.

Enjoy the healing process. There is nothing more important than your health!

---

8. See page 31 for information about how to do enemas.

Mucus Rules

#1 – Avoid eating mucus.

#2 – Mucus-forming foods include meat, dairy, grains, and starches.

#3 – See rule #1.

Peace, Love, and Breath!

Frequently Asked Questions (FAQs) about the Mucusless Diet: An Introduction by Professor Spira

Disclaimer: My views about and experiences with the human body may challenge everything you have been taught. It is necessary for you to free your mind of the many erroneous medical and naturopathic concepts before we get started. Do not just take my word for it. I encourage you to ask questions and research this topic for yourself. The only way that you can truly "know" something is to live and experience it.

Mucusless Diet Healing System
General Introductory Principles

Excerpt based on Lesson I

Every disease, no matter what name it is known by in medical science, is

CONSTIPATION

Constipation is a clogging up of the entire pipe system of the human body with mucus and pus.

Special accumulation points are the tongue, the stomach, and particularly the entire digestive tract. The latter is the real and deeper cause of bowel constipation.

The average person has as much as 10 to 20 pounds of uneliminated feces in their digestive tract. This waste is continually poisoning the bloodstream and the entire body system. Think of it!

Every sick person has a mucus-clogged system derived from undigested, uneliminated, unnatural food substances that have accumulated since childhood.

The *Mucusless Diet Healing System* has proven to be the most successful "compensation action" and so-called "cure" against every type of disease known to mankind.

By its systematic application, thousands of patients that are declared to be incurable could be saved.

BOTH HOW YOU EAT AND WHAT YOU EAT ARE IMPORTANT!

The *Mucusless Diet* consists of all kinds of raw and cooked fruits, starchless vegetables, and cooked or raw mostly green-leaf vegetables.

The *Mucusless Diet Healing System* is a combination of individually advised long- and short-term fasts, menus that progressively change to non-mucus-forming foods, and regular colon irrigation.

This diet alone could heal every case of disease without fasting, although such a cure would require a longer time.

It is a systematic way of eating to transition yourself safely away from disease-producing foods.

FAQs

What are mucus-forming foods?

Dead animal products

Dairy Products

Grains, Starches, and Fats

What do you eat?

I am systematically transitioning my diet to fruits and green-leaf vegetables. Ultimately, these foods will eliminate the need for themselves.

But how do you get protein and vitamins?

I do not believe in the protein theory. The body does not need anything to be a body. You cannot feed protein or anything else to an atom, and we are made up of a bunch of atoms. The body does not get its energy from food or the nutrients found in food. If you break your addiction to so-called "protein (mucus) foods," you will feel much better and see at once how wrong this theory is.

Why do I need colon irrigation?

The human organism is the filthiest being on the planet. No other animal has broken the physiological laws of nature as terribly as humans have. Because of our condition, it is necessary to irrigate our colon regularly to rectify the physiological laws that we and our ancestors have been breaking for thousands of years.

What do you mean by "physiological law"?

I often say that "the world was flat until we realized that it was round." A law is an undeniable truth that is invariable under any given circumstance. Most of us agree on a law called gravity. We agree that if an individual jumps off the top of the Eiffel Tower with no technological apparatus, he or she will fall and die because of the tremendous impact with the ground—due to gravity. This is an example of a "rediscovered" law of which we are all conscious.

In the late 1800s, Professor Arnold Ehret rediscovered the most important, fundamental, and misunderstood universal law regarding human physiology: our bodies are "air-gas engines"! He realized that no matter what we eat, we all run solely on air. He then established the equation, Vitality = Power − Obstruction (V = P - O), to demonstrate this law. Like breaking the law of gravity, if you break this physiological law you will undoubtedly suffer sooner or later. It does not matter whether you disagree with the law, believe in the law, consciously ignore the law, or just not know what it is. You will not be granted a verdict of "not guilty" due to a technicality. It is your duty and privilege to investigate and know the law.

You have the right to stop eating harmful foods. If you give up this right, it will be held against you in accordance with the physiological laws of the universe.

What is meant by V = P - O?

If you were to put sand into the gas chamber of your car, how far do you think your car would go? If your car engine is caked with gunk because you have not had the oil changed in years, how well does the car work? Chances are, it would work much better if gasoline was used instead of sand and the gunk (obstruction) was eliminated with a good oil change. If the basic laws are ignored, the obstruction in the engine becomes too great; the engine cannot function and ultimately stops (dies).

The engine of your body acts in the same way. Your body is an air-gas engine that was never designed to take in food, much less mucus-forming foods. Over time, these mucus-forming foods create so much obstruction that the body can no longer receive efficient amounts of oxygen into the bloodstream. This obstruction is then given some kind of name such as heart attack, stroke, high cholesterol, and so on. To describe this basic principle, Arnold

18

Ehret created the equation, Vitality = Power - Obstruction (i.e., V = P - O). As soon as Obstruction (O) becomes greater than the body's Power (P) deriving from the breath, the body comes to a standstill.

Then what is this eating thing for, if we run on air?

The first thing we must do is humble ourselves, look at ourselves in the mirror, and admit that we are pathologically sick beings addicted to the ultimate gateway drug: pus and mucus. We must eliminate the erroneous medical dogmas that we have been force fed since childhood.

I know that I am addicted to the most insidious drugs that the human body could ever consume: pus and mucus. What can I do about my addiction? I can read the Mucusless Diet Healing System and start to transition away from mucus-forming foods. I can begin to administer lemon enemas to myself regularly and learn how to lie down and fast (refrain from eating solid food) when it is necessary.

The only reason that we eat is to control our bodily elimination.

What about pharmaceutical medications?

The human body is not designed to use the chemicals in medicine whatsoever. Medication is a chemical poison that shocks your body, forcing it to stop its current elimination and deal with the new poison. Therefore, you suppress your current symptoms and go on about your day like everything is normal. Ignoring eliminations through suppression will not make the problem go away. The only way to eliminate what we call sickness is to eliminate mucus from your body and diet.

I thought that Jello was wholesome! Isn't that what they serve sick patients in the hospital?

Jello is made out of ground-up bones, hooves, and other unfortunate parts of animals. Needless to say, it is pure filth and not fit for human consumption, much less hospital patients who desperately need lemon enemas, fruits, vegetables, and prescribed fasts.

How long should I fast?

You must naturally learn how to fast for a long time. As you gain experience, you will learn the length that is right for you. The cleaner your body gets, the easier it will be to fast. Whenever you go through a mucus elimination (get sick), you should immediately stop eating mucus: FAST! If you would like to avoid adding to your current latent sicknesses, then it is advised that the art of fasting be learned without delay.

Just fruits and vegetables?

Mucusless fruits and vegetables are the only foods fit for human consumption. The purpose of eating these foods is to aid the body in its elimination of pus and mucus. While not fasting, fruits and vegetables should be eaten every day. Fruit acts as an aggressive dissolver of mucus, while vegetables function as a mucus broom in the intestines to help the body eliminate the dissolved waste. With that said, in the beginning it may be necessary to eat certain mucus-forming foods to ensure a more comfortable and permanent transition.

What about air and food pollution?

It's interesting when people ask me about surviving as a breathairean[9] in our polluted environment. I look at them and say that we are both standing here surviving exclusively on air right now. Just because I practice the mucusless diet does not mean that my body's operations are any different from the Burger King devotee. The difference is that my operations will not likely be stopped by thick pus in a few years. Food, no matter what it is or how it was grown, is only doing one of two things: it is either adding mucus to the body or eliminating it. I acknowledge that our foods are messed up, but I believe that the concern needs to stay on the food's ability to aid the body's elimination of mucus. Of course, if you are accustomed to organic fruits and vegetables, and can afford them, then I don't see any problem with them. However, I would immediately stop taking any supplements and put that money into big boxes of lemons and distilled water for enemas.

Why doesn't anybody else know about this? Why hasn't this information been on Oprah or 60 Minutes?

Congratulations! You have been given a very rare opportunity indeed. You are one of the first people to be exposed to the most important rediscovery of the twentieth century! We are living in a

---

9. The term "breathairean" refers to an organism whose primary sustenance comes from breathing air.

very degenerate age that may best be described as the latter part of the Middle Ages. A time when death and the eating of death is deemed to be totally normal! We are all a part of a worldwide death culture that is dedicated to chaos, ignorance, and self-degeneration.

As Gil Scott-Heron said, "THE REVOLUTION WILL NOT BE TELEVISED!" Since Ehret's rediscovery in the late 1800s, pioneering individuals in the United States and Europe have continued his work and are the living examples of its truth. Thousands of people from Italy and elsewhere have formed mucusless communities. These people are all vessels of real human knowledge. As Brother Air says, "If you do not know how your body operates, you can be told anything."

Since Ehret's rediscovery, media controllers have done everything in their power to suppress the work of Arnold Ehret and other naturopaths. Every day, we are bombarded with erroneous health information and are bamboozled into believing that we do not control 100 percent of our health through what we put into our bodies. The implications and acceptance of Ehret's work would ultimately lead to the abolition of the medical, meat, and dairy industries, among others. Eventually, the current system of capitalism would be rendered useless and the Earth's people would return back to the mythical "Garden of Eden," one of the universal paradise myths shared by many divergent cultures.

But I love to eat! I don't think that I could ever stop eating. It tastes too good. I love food with a passion. You are wrong, you have to be, right? Shouldn't a diet be well balanced? Eating is a part of my culture and heritage, and I refuse be preached to!

I am in no way, shape, or form telling you to just stop eating. I'm not preaching about what is good and bad for you, or what you should believe in. I am a humble musician, professor, philosopher, and mucusless diet practitioner with the obligation to share these newly rediscovered laws with you. I am challenging you with profound information that has the power to transform your life. Only you can transform this information into knowledge and evolve it into wisdom. My words mean nothing unless you decide to be proactive and investigate these principles for yourself. No matter what you decide to do, you have been chosen to receive this information NOW. And right NOW, armed with the knowledge of these physiological laws, you have a wonderful opportunity to question and investigate the limitless potential of the human body.

What is inside of us?

¡Mucus!

¡Mucus!

¡Mucus!

What is there to eat to help eliminate this waste?

Fruits and green, leafy vegetables

Peace, Love, and Breath!

-Prof. Spira

Biography of Arnold Ehret by Prof. Spira

By 2006, the online, user-driven encyclopedia Wikipedia was becoming more and more popular. Many of the most important and influential historical figures already had thorough biographies. Yet, whenever I searched for Arnold Ehret, there was no biography to be found. I decided to take it upon myself to review various sources and create his first substantial Wikipedia biography. I also scanned the famous picture of Ehret I had, added some red colored saturation effects to it, and submitted it as the original picture. In the following years, Ehret grew in popularity and the Wikipedia site seemed to be the first stop for many seeking information about his work. Also, the biography that I originally wrote was translated into various languages through Wikipedia and accessed by people around the world.

Although my biography was basic, I had hoped that others would come along and improve it, adding more critical analyses and pertinent details. That is exactly what has happened! Today, Arnold Ehret's Wikipedia biography[10] is fairly comprehensive and substantial. I am very proud to have contributed to the evolution of this source, which has become many health seekers' first introduction to the monumental works of Prof. Arnold Ehret.

Below is my original biography. Sources include writings about Ehret by Fred Hirsch and Gordon Kennedy, as well as personal memoirs by Ehret embedded into his dietetic writings.

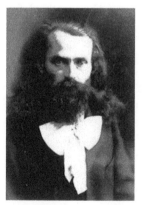

Professor Arnold Ehret, revered as the father of naturopathy, is one of the most important pioneering researchers and authors regarding the health and preservation of the human body. No other scientist, doctor, dietitian, or author has surpassed Ehret's work concerning the cause and cure of chronic disease and human illness. Through years of research, he rediscovered that the human body is an "air-gas engine" that is powered exclusively by oxygen, and that a diet consisting of starchless fruits and green, leafy vegetables is the only food fit for human consumption. Among other important writings, Ehret produced a brilliant dietetic treatise entitled The *Mucusless Diet Healing System*, which

---

10. See http://en.wikipedia.org/wiki/Arnold_Ehret.

offers a methodical approach to eating that can be used regardless of age, gender, race, or sickness to achieve superior health.

Arnold Ehret was born July 29, 1866, near Freiburg, in Baden, Germany. His father was a brilliant farmer who was so technologically advanced that he crafted his own farming equipment. Like his father, Ehret would be endowed with a passion for studying the cause and effect of phenomena. His courses of interest were physics, chemistry, drawing, and painting. He also had an affinity for linguistics and could speak German, French, Italian, and English. At the age of 21, he graduated as a professor of drawing and was drafted into the military, only to be discharged because of heart trouble. At the age of 31, he was diagnosed with Bright's disease (inflammation of the kidneys) and pronounced incurable by 24 of Europe's most respected doctors. He then explored natural healing and visited sanitariums to learn holistic methods and philosophies. In a desperate attempt to quench his misery, Ehret decided to stop eating. To his amazement, he did not die but gained in strength and vitality.

In 1899, he traveled to Berlin to study vegetarianism, followed by a trip to Algiers in northern Africa where he experimented with fasting and fruit dieting. As a result of his new lifestyle, Ehret cured himself of all of his illnesses and could then perform great feats of physiological strength, including an 800-mile bicycle trip from Algiers to Tunis. His findings led him to cultivate the "Mucus Theory," which explains how pus- and mucus-forming foods are the cause of all human disease, and that "fasting" (simply eating less) is Nature's omnipotent method for cleansing the body from the effects of wrong food choices and too much eating.[11]

In the early 1900s, Ehret opened a hugely popular sanitarium in Ascona, Switzerland where he treated and cured thousands of patients considered incurable by the so-called "medical authorities." During the latter part of the decade, Ehret engaged in a series of fasts monitored by German and Swiss officials. Within a period of 14 months, Ehret completed one fast of 21 days, one of 24 days, one of 32 days, and one of 49 days. The latter remained the world record for many decades. He became one of the most in-demand health lecturers, journalists, and

11. Hirsch, Fred, "Introduction," in *Arnold Ehret's Mucusless Diet Healing System: A Complete Course for Those Who Desire to Learn How to Control Their Health* (Dobbs Ferry, NY: Ehret Literature, 1994), 9.

educators in Europe, saving the lives of thousands of people. In 1914, Ehret moved his sanitarium to California and championed his *Mucusless Diet Healing System* in America.

On October 9, 1922, at the age of 56, Arnold Ehret suffered a tragic fall and sustained a fatal blow to his skull. According to his disciple Fred Hirsch, Ehret was walking briskly on a wet, oil-soaked street during foggy conditions when he slipped and fell backward onto his head. Hirsch did not actually see the fall but found Ehret lying on the street. Another of Ehret's disciples, Benedict Lust, maintained that Ehret was wearing his first pair of new dress shoes and slipped as a result of his unfamiliarity with the footwear.[12] To this day, the true nature of Ehret's death raises many suspicions among Ehretists. Ehret's powerful healing successes, along with his influential and revolutionary new lifestyle, terribly threatened the medical, meat, and dairy industries. Due to these factors, many believe that foul play was involved in Ehret's untimely death.

Arnold Ehret is a cultural icon and was an important protagonist of the emerging back-to-nature renaissance in Germany and Switzerland during the latter part of the nineteenth century.[13] The influence of this renaissance spread to America and influenced many of the counter-cultural movements including the beat generation, the vegetarian-driven "hippie" movement, veganism, and fruitarianism. Throughout the twentieth and into the twenty-first centuries, the teachings of Ehret have thrived and developed through the sincere efforts of a small group of dedicated Ehretists. Today, Ehret's teachings are gaining wider acceptance throughout the world as people discover for themselves the undeniable truth of his teachings.

---

12. Ehret, Arnold, *Mucusless Diet Healing System [MDHS] a Scientific Method of Eating Your Way to Health, with Introduction by Benedict Lust* (New York: Benedict Lust Publishers, 1970 [2002]), page preceding i.

13. Kennedy, Gordon, "Arnold Ehret," in *Children of the Sun: A Pictorial Anthology, from Germany to California: 1883-1949*, 144-153 (Ojai, CA: Nivaria Press, 1998). (Also see Kennedy's article, "Hippie Roots & the Perennial Subculture.")

Chapter 2—The Ehret Health Club Correspondence

Introduction

The following chapters contain my first writings about the *Mucusless Diet Healing System*. These articles were initially published on the Ehret Health Club website administered by Alvin Last, the former owner of Ehret Publishing. My intention was to connect with other people interested in Arnold Ehret's work and share the news of our movement toward Physiological Liberation. In particular, I wanted to inform them of the important contributions by Cincinnati's Ehretist community and answer general questions.

Greetings Brothers and Sisters!

Posted on December 19, 2005 by Professor Spira

My name is Professor Spira. I live in Cincinnati, Ohio and am pursuing a master's degree in jazz trombone performance at the College-Conservatory of Music, University of Cincinnati. I started practicing the *Mucusless Diet Healing System* about 3 ½ years ago. Since then, I lost over 120 pounds—I used to be a 280-pound football player—and cured all of my ailments, including chronic migraine headaches, lower back pain, joint pain in my right hand ("from football" but really just from mucus), chronic pain in my right knee, chronic allergies, and otolaryngological problems including chronic cases of bronchitis. I was emancipated forever of the numerous pharmaceuticals that I had been taking since I was 7 years old, as well as addictions to tobacco and alcohol. I also was able to do away with a CPAP unit (a machine that pumps oxygen into constipated, sleeping noses) for my bad case of "Sleep Apnea." I definitely consider myself a Mucusless Diet success story.

I found out about the diet from a jazz musician in Cincinnati who goes by the name Brother Air. Brother Air has been practicing the diet for about 25 years. In fact, Cincinnati is thriving with people who practice the *Mucusless Diet*. I am thankful to have had the good fortune of being around people who practice the diet on a high level, which enabled me to ask many questions and see firsthand what the diet is all about. I was very impressed with Brother Air's stories of sustaining an all-fruit diet for an entire year, but nothing was more impressive than witnessing him do an 8½-month juice fast. Seeing a man fast with such ease for that length of time shattered any doubt I had about humans' potential to become fruitarians and beyond. Despite the short amount of time I had spent transitioning, I started a fast in January of 2005 and ended in July. I followed it gracefully with an all-fruit diet, then vegetables [I have still not returned to eating every day yet, and hope that I do not have to]. I did not try to fast for 6 months, it was just the logical conclusion of the rigorous physiological work that I had been doing. The interesting thing about my fast was that it was done while I was earning my bachelor's degree at CCM. My peers were amazed at my physiological changes, and that I did not look emaciated. Others in our Ehretist community witnessed my fasting and were inspired themselves, including the violinist Loving Star who recently juice fasted for 35 days.

The key to all of our successes is a proper transition with the systematic use of enemas. The *Mucusless Diet Healing System* practitioners in our camp all do lemon-juice enemas almost every day. Despite Ehret's somewhat passive language as it pertains to enemas, we have found it essential to bring out the full potential of the diet. For the first 3 months, I did not do enemas; I received some decent results, but was still having troubling kicking meat. As soon as I started doing lemon juice enemas, with transitional menus, the old meat poisons were eliminated, as well as heavy starch cravings. (Nothing feels better than fasting for about a week and then doing an enema that eliminates about 3 pounds of stringy fecal matter that smells like rotten eggs.)

Cincinnati is also the home of the all-vegetarian and Ehretist band Breathairean Ensemble, which is a band consisting mostly of individuals pursuing a mucusless lifestyle. The band acts as a support system for its members as we practice the diet. Musically, the band is influenced by such artists as John Coltrane, Sun Ra, and the Art Ensemble of Chicago. We perform music pieces that are inspired by the *Mucusless Diet Healing System*, many of which contain dialog about the diet and our philosophies. Our mission is to spread the good news to the world through vibrations of discipline, beauty, and cleanliness.

I have numerous stories that may be of interest to others who believe in Ehret's teachings and I would love to share them. At first, I was a bit reluctant to write because I am not looking for any adversarial energy. I know that many of you may believe in some of the theories of "so-called" medical science or are confused about what to believe, and I respect this whole heartedly. I, myself, do not believe in the protein theory, vitamin theory, or the standard nutrition theories propagated by medical scientists. I do not think that the body can, or needs to, absorb and assimilate the dead elements found in dead foods for the purposes of gaining energy (the additive principle). Yet, the body uses food primarily for the purpose of eliminating pus, mucus, and toxemias from the bloodstream (unless it is mucus-forming food, then it is assimilated into the tissue system to later become illness). I view the body as an air-gas engine that is primarily fueled by the air we breathe.

About fasting, it must be said that I would never tell somebody to stop eating, nor would I recommend a long fast. In fact, after my extended fasts, I had to give many lectures to frustrated practitioners on the importance of a proper transition before any fasting cures. I stress a proper transitional diet along with enemas and patience. The diet must be embraced as a lifestyle in order to achieve the superior health spoken of by Ehret. Only through long-term practice can one hope to avoid disease and suffering.

Peace, Love, and Breath!

-Professor Spira

Responses

Posted on December 19, 2005 by Kim

I am amazed at your story. You really give hope to us all. Hope to hear more from you on a regular basis.

-Kim Raylee

Posted on December 19, 2005 by Divine Scientist

Good teaching, Professor! Very inspirational! Kindly share the wealth of your knowledge and experience. This isn't an adversarial forum, but one where we can share experience, knowledge and inspiration!

-Divine Scientist

Posted on December 21, 2005 by Thank You Arnold/Wader

Yes, welcome! Please share the wealth in your health and your road to getting there. Also, any other experiences/knowledge is indeed welcome!

Satan is a very busy individual, both in confusing biblical truth and confusing the road to successful (as well as many other things), paradisiac health. It would be a pleasure to read the writing of a current individual's road/path to success. How did they start, what did they do to transition (foods-types/kinds, fasts-how long/often, type drinks/fluids, enemas—as you've already described, etc.).

There are so many different ideas, theories, etc. out there beyond what Arnold achieved, which only confuse the road to a successful result. So, indeed, it would be deeply appreciated to read your detailed road to success with this diet.

I started this diet on October 29th of this year. I was suffering from fibromyalgia and narcolepsy. My fibromyalgia symptoms disappeared within 2 weeks and the narcolepsy is subsiding. My spouse started a couple of weeks later. She too, suffers from arthritis, among other things.

Our teenage son began shortly after that, fell back after about 2 weeks for 1 week, and then returned to the diet again. We still have many questions and much learning to do. It would be wonderful to hear from an experienced individual who has achieved the very success we are looking for.

Please, share all you can and feel comfortable with, as I know our family would deeply appreciate it and learn from the information, direction and/or details you provide.

Thank you for being here and taking the time to post!

First question we have is how much/kind of lemon juice mix is put in the enemas? What's the formula?

God bless!

-Thank You Arnold/Tim Wader

The All-Important Lemon Enema

Posted on December 23, 2005 by Professor Spira

I cannot say enough about the lemon enema! Brother Air started doing lemon enemas in the 1980s and witnessed how much more effective they were than distilled water. He saw and felt significant changes immediately, and has done lemon enemas exclusively ever since. Today, he juices anywhere from 5 to 25 lemons in a citrus juicer and uses warm distilled water. I also started my lemon enema journey using about 5 lemons with a citrus juicer. A little way down the road, I obtained a Jack LaLanne juicer and started peeling the lemons and using that. This made the enemas much more potent. Then, I started juicing the whole lemon and filtering out some of the grit. One day, I decided to try it without straining the grit and found my new best friend, what I call the Lemon Rind Enema. Once I started doing enemas like this, the old citrus juicer-style enema was like doing water enemas. I attribute a great deal of my personal success with the system thus far to the Lemon Rind Enema.

For those of you who may be interested in dabbling with the lemon enema, I suggest a TRANSITION. I did not get to the point where I could hold 25 lemons in for 20 minutes all at once. Start with the juice of a couple lemons combined with warm water. You want enough lemons so that you can feel it breaking down the mucus on the walls of your intestines, but not so potent that you cannot hold it in for any length of time.

Question: What if I cannot hold my enemas very long? What should I do? Holding in the lemons for a shorter amount of time is totally normal. Any discomfort that you feel is due to the lemon acid breaking down the pools of mucus lining your intestines. The longer you do them, the easier it will become to hold it in longer if you desire. I've found that the length of time you hold it in is not as important as the amount of times [frequency] that you do it. I would much rather see someone do two 3-minute enemas with heavy lemon than one 30-minute water enema. Think of your intestine as a pipe. When you cut a 30-year-old kitchen pipe that has never been cleaned and study it, you can see layers of caked-on debris. The closer you get to the metal inside of the pipe, the older and tougher the deposits are. To clean it, you can submerge it into a solvent and then scrub out the loosened debris. However, our intestines are not metal, but are composed of soft tissues. The *Mucusless Diet* and fasting gives your system a rest, allowing the intestinal walls to

31

secrete these layers of mucus/debris that have accumulated during your lifetime. The citric acid from the lemons assail the adhesive properties of the slime, enabling it to either come out immediately or be flushed out later by another enema. When one layer is eliminated, a whole new layer is now waiting to be loosened and eliminated. Every time the mucus is exposed to the lemon acid, its adhesive properties are diminished, therefore making the amount of lemon enemas that you do more important than how long you hold them in (since holding them in for longer periods will come in time anyway). And the astringent properties of the lemon will pull on the lining of the intestines, allowing for cleansing beyond the outside of the intestinal wall. Now you may understand why long fasts or long fruit/raw diets are ineffective to a filthy body. Eating fruit loosens the mucus, the vegetables act as a broom sweeping the garbage to the colonic dust bin, and the enema helps empty the garbage. Fasting then becomes the result of a less-obstructed body: Vitality = Power - Obstruction . What a perfect system!

Question: Won't I become addicted to enemas or overstimulate my colon? From my own experience and from the testimony of others I know, the bowels work much better while doing regular enemas. I have no problem having natural bowel movements and often have them before doing my enema. Also, distilled water—or distilled water and lemon juice—is not harmful to the colon or system. I never advocate any other kind of enema, such as coffee or Fleet, because they are detrimental to your system. Coffee, or as Brother Air calls it, "bean soup," is a stimulant and has no cleansing properties. When initiating a cleansing diet or fast, I would say that colon irrigation is of the utmost importance. As you begin to systematically loosen the waste in your gastrointestinal tract, enemas will be exceedingly helpful in removing harmful toxic waste in a timely fashion. In fact, it is dangerous to have such waste circulating in your system. After the initial periods of cleansing, regular use of enemas may be viewed as general hygiene. As long as we are eating mucus-forming foods or have constitutional encumbrances in our system, performing regular colon irrigation will be useful and not harmful.

Question: Should I get a colonic instead? This form of colon irrigation can be very useful, especially during or following a fast. Yet, I view colonics as a specific kind of tool/therapy that need not replace or be equated to enemas. In my opinion, nothing beats consistent enemas performed regularly over a long time. Also, self-prepared enemas give you the opportunity to add lemon juice. But, if you have the means to get a professionally administered colonic, or experiment with a colema board at your home, I encourage you to do so. Yet, I would strongly encourage you to not substitute colonics for regular lemon enemas but synthesize the two irrigation tools.

Here is my step-by-step enema process:

Instructions

1. Obtain an enema/douche bag/hot water bottle system (often found at medical supply stores or in feminine-hygiene departments in supermarkets and drug stores. Make sure to get the enema system and not *only* the hot water bottle).

2. Obtain lemons. I buy boxes of lemons from a local wholesaler. (Note: Do not use bottled, store bought lemon juice.)

3. Obtain distilled water.

4. Find out how much water/juice will be necessary by filling the bag and pouring the water back into a container for measurement. When filled, mine holds a little over 1.5 liters.

5. Prepare the enema bag by attaching one side of the tubing to the adapter cap, thread the clamp, and allow it to remain near the opposite end. Finally, insert the anal piece to the end opposite of the adapter cap.

6. Juice the lemons. I started off juicing three or four lemons with a citrus juicer and eventually moved to juicing eight to ten whole lemons with the rind. Once I started doing lemon rind enemas, I realized that I had found a truly wonderful key for healing the human organism. However, if you are concerned about pesticides, or if it is too potent, just cut off the skin or use a citrus juicer. (Note: lime juice can be used when lemons are too expensive or hard to find.)

7. Combine the necessary amount of distilled water with the lemon juice. (Note: if you find lemon enemas to be too aggressive, then just do distilled water enemas with half of a squeezed lemon or without lemon juice. Even the juice from half of a lemon can be beneficial.)

8. Heat the combination on the stove. The water should not be scalding, but good and warm. The warmer the better!

9. Put the warmed water/juice in the enema bag.

10. Find a cozy place near the toilet to lie down. I use an old Boy Scout ground cloth, thick towel, and pillow on the ground in the hall outside of my small bathroom. If the bathroom is big enough, you can lie in there. (In the college dormitories, I did them in a public restroom that could lock from the inside—there are many fun stories that I can tell you about that later!)

11. Use your choice of lubricant on the tip of the anal piece and your hind parts.

12. Allow a small amount of the water to shoot into the sink from your enema bag and then use the clamp to stop the water flow. (Brother Air does not use a clamp but just tilts the tube upward and uses gravity until he is ready.)

13. Lie down on your back and gently massage your stomach and intestines. Take some deep breaths and relax. This is meant to be a relaxing, stress-free therapy. This is an opportunity to release your body from the buildup of unnecessary internal waste. (Optionally, light incense or candles, listen to music, have reading materials near—wonderful to do with Ehret's books.)

14. *What side to lie on?* There is some debate about what side is best to lie on while injecting the liquid during an enema. Some literature says that lying on your right side allows gravity to help the water effectively enter the intestines; others say that the left is best. When I started, I layed on my right side, but now I lie on my left. I've tried both sides—each works and seems to have their own advantages. I'm currently doing my enemas on my left side.

15. After you lie down on your side, relax and gently insert the anal piece.

16. There are several ways to allow the water to flow from the bag. I usually hold the bag in my hand and gently squeeze it. I might also raise the bag up with my hand and let gravity cause the water to flow. Another method is to use a metal rod with a spiral curve at the end to raise the bag higher in the air. Also, some people use a pear-shaped enema bag hook (or shower curtain hook) that can be attached to a shower rod, door handle, or IV stand. The speed and

flow of the water can be controlled by how high you choose to elevate the bag, how hard you squeeze, or by applying and releasing pressure using the clip or your fingers on the tube.

17. Once the water is inside your intestines, hold it in as long as you can. After a while, perhaps a minute or two, you may shift to lying on your back. Later, you may eventually shift to the side opposite the one that you were on to insert the water. You can also tilt your body upward to allow gravity to bring the water down as far as possible. Brother Air uses a yogic position where he stands on his head, sometimes for extended periods of time. I never learned to stand on my head, but I usually am able to tilt my body up so that it is on an incline. While in the dorms, I would prop my feet against the wall and allow the middle part of my body to be close to a 90-degree angle with the floor.

18. After a certain time, you will feel the need to evacuate the water. Sit on the toilet and let the waste drain from you. You may periodically gently massage your intestines as you sit. Sometimes I will eliminate a portion and then return to my ground cloth to lie down for several more minutes. How long it will take before you feel the need to eliminate depends upon how much waste you have in your intestines and how experienced you are with performing enemas. I usually hold it in from 5 to 15 minutes; while Brother Air might hold his for 30 to 45 minutes or even longer. (Do not be deterred by Brother Air, as he may be viewed as the *Michael Jordan* of this healing modality.) Since I tend to make my lemon water more potent through juicing the rind and all, I usually eliminate a bit quicker. With that said, sometimes you will feel the need to eliminate immediately, or even after only putting in half of the water from your bag. Either way, it is all beneficial. (Note: in the beginning, you may actually put the water in and not see much come back out. If this happens, the water is absorbing into the years of caked on filth in your intestines. After a series of days or weeks with consistent lemon enemas, eventually you may be surprised by a huge elimination where large amounts of loosened waste are evacuated at once.)

19. Take some deep breaths and smile, as you have taken one more step toward physiological liberation!

20. Peace, Love, and Breath!

SEE?

Squeeze me out
Heat me up
Then shoot me up and let me go to work.

If you could only see what I see,
YEARS of caked-on
FILTH!

It's my job to help clean it up.
I'll help loosen this mess
as much as I can.

Uh-oh, that's enough, time to shoot back out!

SEE?

That wasn't so bad,
And I may have just saved your life,
For I am the all-important lemon enema.

-Prof. Spira

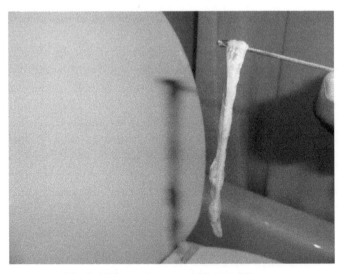

Muciod Plaque from one of Spira's Enemas

36

Prof. Arnold Ehret on Enemas

Quotes from *Rational Fasting for Physical, Mental, & Spiritual Rejuvenation:*

"In spite of the above, every cure, and especially every cure of diet, should start with a 2- or 3-day fast. Every patient can do this without any harm, regardless of how seriously sick he may be. First a laxative and then an enema daily makes it easier as well as harmless."

"First—Prepare for an easier fast by a gradually changing diet toward a mucusless diet, and natural herbal laxatives and enemas."

"Rules During the Fast: 1. Clean the lower intestines as well as you can with enemas at least every other day."

"During a fast, and even during the "transition period," the bowel evacuation contains sticky, stringy mucus difficult for normal elimination, and it is here that enemas prove helpful."

"If it is not desired to take a more prolonged fast, although he is healthy, one should try a short one. Even a fasting of 36 hours weekly, one or two times, can be depended upon to produce very favorable results. It is best to start by leaving off the supper and taking an enema instead."

"If no good stool is experienced after 2 or 3 hours, help with laxatives and enemas. Whenever I fasted, I always experienced a good bowel movement at least 1 hour after eating and at once felt fine. After breaking a long fast, I spent more time on the toilet than in bed the following night—and that was as it should be."

"If any extraordinary sensation occurs due to the drugs that are now in circulation, take an enema at once, lie down, and if necessary break the fast but not with fruits."

"Air baths taken in the room, enemas, laxatives, and cool lemonade would save the lives of thousands of young men and women who are now daily permitted to die, the innocent victims of pneumonia or other acute diseases, due to the stubborn ignorance of doctors and so-called highly civilized people."

More on enemas in this book: Ehret's Intestinal Broom vs. Enemas (p. 61), Enemas and Social Dissonances (p. 62), Never Too Early to Begin Enemas (p. 85), Where to Get Enema Supplies (p. 86), Doing Enemas in a House Filled with People (p. 86), Doing Daily Enemas and Questions about the 80/10/10 Diet (p. 176)

Clearing Up Myths with Experience, Part 1

Posted on December 23, 2005 by Thank You Prof. Ehret/Wader

Hi Spira! Haha! That was too funny! Valuable and true, but funny! Completely enjoyed that! Thanks so much for the details on the *lemona's* (our new name for them). That was very deeply appreciated. We will be starting those immediately! I would definitely agree on the transition. That would be a high amount to start with. Does your juicer actually break down the rinds that well? Or are you talking about just the pulp (without the strainer in the juicer)? We have an Acme juicer.

It sounds like you're in a perfect area of the country for the diet. We only know of one individual here who has been on it for about 3 years. There is a lot to learn, especially about transitioning. I personally don't have alcohol to deal with, but unfortunately, I do have tobacco and coffee. I plan on eliminating at least one by the end of this year. They are already beginning to be a turnoff as Arnold mentioned they would.

Breathairean, how perfect! We are so proud of you and pass on how proud we are of all those around you succeeding in the diet, achieving such incredible success! Our goal is to never give up on the diet, continually learn and succeed to the level of health you are speaking of. Again, we are sure we have a lot to learn. Thank you for being here, offering an experienced, successful level of assistance for all of us who want to reach the level you and others have reached in Cincinnati. You have no idea how deeply appreciated your presence here is.

When you mentioned transitional menus, would you recommend those spoken of in *Live Foods*? We have been doing the first 2-month menus which Arnold detailed out in the *Mucusless Diet Healing System* book, but have been trying to plan what direction to take after that. He also mentioned some other menu items too. Some of the items mentioned in these books seem to be against what Arnold spoke of: high in proteins, etc., things like that. So, sometimes confusing. I'm sure it's just a lack of knowledge on our part at this point. Any assistance you could provide☺ in this area as well would be immensely appreciated.

Again, Spira, thanks for being here and God Bless! It is a pleasure hearing from you! Have a wonderful, peaceful, healthy, and Happy Holiday!!

God Bless

TYA

P.S. I know you mentioned not being in favor of vitamins, but what about the quality of the foods out there today? Studies have shown how much of the vegetables, etc., out there are coming in at up to 50 percent lower levels of vitamins, minerals, etc. We've been on the Garden of Life, Perfect Food organic, whole food, non-isolated, non-synthetic supplement due to that concern and that of B-12.

Any thoughts or knowledge in that area as well? Our family thanks you SO much in advance, over and over again!

-Thank You Prof. Ehret/Wader

Spira's Response

Posted on December 25, 2005 by Professor Spira

My Jack LaLanne Juicer does an excellent job with juicing the whole lemon. I peel the skin off when I plan to drink citrus juice, but for my enema purposes the peel breaks down to make the juice really thick and potent. Despite its thickness, the liquid flows through the hose free of obstruction.

I have not thoroughly read the *Live Foods* book yet. I believe that I may have paged through it in a health-food store only to put it down when it said some irrational things. You may be able to get some ideas out of the book, but I've always tried to keep things as simple as possible. After practicing the weekly transitional menus provided by Ehret for a while, I moved into a menu that usually consisted of a fruit meal at lunchtime and a big salad with some steamed vegetables (usually broccoli and cabbage) with toasted wheat bread for dinner, followed much later by some fruit juice. On a day when I crave some mucus, I will attack the craving with some of the mucus-lean menus out of the book or the ones recommended to me by my colleagues. One approach that I learned was to try to focus on staying mucusless for extended periods of time. Many people try to do long fasts or fruit/raw fasts, but I would love to hear people say things like, "I did a month totally mucusless." Even though I went 6 months without eating any solid food, for me the real accomplishment was going 9 months totally mucusless.

Others have asked me what I do to create a variety in my meals. I say that I really try to go long stretches on one thing. Once I find a nice groove, I try to wear it out. For instance, the past week I have made the same pineapple-strawberry-banana-blueberry juice every day. I may add or subtract a different kind of fruit next week and that will make it feel like a totally different meal.

If you do venture outside of the Ehret book to look for ideas, just try to monitor your selections. Avoid going down roads that will lead you to physiological dead ends. The doctrine that I base my life around is the **"need principle**." Before I do anything, I ask myself if I truly need it.

"Do I need this piece of pineapple? Yes, because I have mucus in me that needs to be loosened."

"Do I need these nuts today? No, physiologically, I think I can do without them right now."

Furthermore, I am constantly preparing myself psychologically for every physiological advance. I refuse to let the obstruction in my mind keep me from reaching my full potential on the diet. Our culture revolves around the "additive principle." It is drilled into our heads since birth that our bodies need foreign things to be bodies. We are led to believe that if our body does not receive the correct substances, we will have problems. OUR BODIES ARE AIR-GAS ENGINES THAT RUN ON AIR EXCLUSIVELY! Think about it. All these years that we have been eating, we have thought it was the food that was keeping us going. However, it doesn't matter if you are in McDonald's drive-through or the health-food store; you are running exclusively on air. Then what is this eating thing for, if we are air-gas engines? Well, unfortunately, the tissue systems of our bodies are permeated with mucus and we are addicted to stimulants (foods) that will add to this mucus. The good news is that we know about a dietary system that, when practiced correctly, allows the body to safely eliminate this mucus, thereby liberating it from its addictions to stimulants/food.

It's interesting when people ask me about surviving as a breathairean (i.e., air eater) in our polluted environment. I look at them and say that we are both standing here, surviving exclusively on air right now. Just because I practice the diet does not mean that my body's operations are any different from the *Burger King* devotee. The difference is that my operations will probably not be stopped by thick pus in a few years. Food, no matter what it is or how it was grown, is only doing one of two things: it is either adding mucus to the body or eliminating it. I acknowledge that our foods are messed up, but I believe that the concern needs to stay on the elimination of mucus. Of course, if you are accustomed to organic fruits and vegetables and can afford them, then I don't see any problem with them. However, I would immediately stop taking any supplements and put that money into big boxes of lemons.

Peace, Love, and Breath!

-Prof. Spira

Clearing Up Myths with Experience, Part 2

Posted on December 25, 2005 by the Wader Family

Hi Spira! Happy Holidays! First, I must say, thanks for the internet! It is a very nice, comforting feeling to be able to communicate with someone who has been successful with this diet, able to keep it simple, and answer questions. It must be great to be living in an area where you have those around you who have succeeded in the diet. Here, at least around us, there is indeed an abundance of naysayers, but then there is also an abundance of customers for the medical profession as well.

I was happy to read your reply about what direction to take menu-wise after the first 2 months. We were actually thinking of doing the same, but wanted some assurance from someone with successful experience. That is a great idea on how to handle the cravings. Fortunately, so far anyway, the cravings haven't really hit me. They have hit my spouse and son, though. We would also have to agree with your comments on the *Live Foods* book. We found some of the comments in there sort of off–base, really, in comparison with Arnold's writings. We did carefully go through the book and marked items that we felt were in agreement with Arnold. We are trying, as you stated, to keep it simple, but having the lack of experienced, successful knowledge around us can make it difficult at times.

That made total sense, what you wrote though about the air-gas engine. Why would the body really need anything else if in perfect working condition? It appeared even that God, in the Garden of Eden, wanted food for man to be a pleasure and not so much a necessity. Even when he brought Adam to life, it stated that He breathed the *breath* of life into him and not the *food* of life. We were basically vegetarian prior to this diet, and the whole food supplement came to us in reading a lot of information about the lack of B-12 in vegetarian, fruitarian diets. So, to be sure the blood builder, energy builder was there, we started the supplements. As far as I understand it though, our bodies provide their own B-12, using very, very small amounts and actually reabsorb it for later use. Do you have any knowledge/information on that? I would agree with the diverting of the funds to lemons, though. We started the lemonas and I know that I can certainly feel a difference in the workings of the enema. I believe it is making a significant difference in the effectiveness. Thank you for that information and knowledge sharing.

On the need principle—great principle by the way—when you said I know I have mucus in me that needs to be loosened, are you using the "magic mirror" to determine that? Also, are you selective in which kinds of nuts you eat? We were wondering about this because our family loves a huge variety of nuts, but have been trying really hard to stick with those that are closer to neutral acid forming. I kind of remember Arnold saying somewhere that black pepper was not a good thing to use, but isn't it basically a dried fruit and if pure, what are your thoughts on using it? What are the thoughts there on pure honey, pure maple syrup, and maple sugar (dry and/or creamy), because we remember Arnold saying that sugars are mucus-forming. Do you have Expos, meetings, fairs, or conventions on the diet there, where people who are on the diet, beginning the diet, or interested can gather for support, information, Q&A's? We haven't seen or heard much about the diet here where we live.

Well, I hope we didn't ask too much or overload with our post. It is truly a Godsend to have you here on the board to share the knowledge and experiences of success from yourself and those around you. It is indeed a pleasure and a blessing to be able to chat with you here.

Again Spira, thank you so much for being here and making yourself available to us who are very thirsty for direction, information, and answers, and have a deep desire to fully succeed in this diet. Thank you!

God Bless, TYA

-Thank You Arnold/Wader

Spira's Response:

Posted on December 26, 2005 by Professor Spira

People, in a sick and pathological state, developed all of these erroneous theories about vitamins and proteins. This explains why the medical establishment is fundamentally flawed beyond repair. When it comes to health, the medical and holistic worlds both insist that your body needs something to operate properly. Through experimentation, they figure out how certain formulas of chemical compounds react with the body. They notice how a certain compound seems to "cure" a certain ailment. Unfortunately, the so-called scientists who perform these experiments do not really have a clue as to how their bodies operate. If they knew, then they would understand why a dog that is fed

43

only water would die before a dog fed only flour and water mixture would—based on Francois Magendie's experiment that resulted in the creation of the protein theory. The dog that is fed just water eliminates much too fast! It is such a filthy organism that it actually needs to eat mucus-forming foods to slow down the elimination, to prevent it from drowning in its own waste.

The area of the medical world that I have great respect for is that of trauma. If someone gets into a tragic car crash or needs an arm reattached, then the emergency room is the best place for them. However, necessity is the mother of invention as far as the trauma unit is concerned, and mucus is definitely to thank for their existence. If you take pus and mucus out of the equation, you would not have a bunch of lunatics running around putting themselves in situations where their bodies would be in jeopardy. Brother Air often asked me to imagine a meeting with a room full of breathairean or fruitarian leaders. If somebody came to them with an idea about building an object that would pollute the AIR and transport humans by hurling them down hard pavement, that person would be forcibly given a 50-lemon colonic and put into a padded room to fast for a few weeks.

Whenever we are provoked by the erroneous concepts that we have been programmed to respect since childhood, we must have courage in the unknown. Simple logic will always save the day. I know plenty of pus- and mucus-eaters who have suffered and died from disease, but I do not know anybody who died eating only fruits and green-leaf vegetables. In this equation, the potential that is found in the unknown seems like a logical path to trod, as opposed to the undeniable fact that if you eat pus and mucus, you will suffer great illness and die.

The following quote is from Wikipedia about the origin of Vitamin B-12:

> B-12 deficiency is the cause of several forms of anemia. The treatment for this disease was first devised by William Murphy who bled dogs to make them anemic and then fed them various substances to see what (if anything) would make them healthy again. He discovered that ingesting large amounts of liver seemed to cure the disease. George Minot and George Whipple then set about to chemically isolate the curative substance and ultimately were able to isolate Vitamin B-12

44

from the liver. For this, all three shared the 1934 Nobel Prize in Medicine.[14]

Check out this madness. Murphy reasoned that pus helped save an anemic dog from certain death. Twisted and absurd! Experiments of this nature could only be conceived of by a completely sick and vile creature (I use the word crEATure because it contains the word EAT). It is time for us to put our faith in our own bodies and experiences. The days of sick, bald creatures in white labcoats telling us about health are over. We are the scientists and the authorities on how the human body operates because we are the ones doing the work.

In regards to vegetarianism and anemia, the sickness does not have anything to do with not receiving all of the goodness that livers and chickens provide, but the heavy starch intake in the mucus-vegetarian's diet promotes an overflow of harmful dead white blood into the body (obstruction/mucus). The misconception often derives from typical mucus-vegetarians who become sickly and die faster than one-sided meat eaters do, due to the morbid amounts of starches that they are consuming. Under the law, the body with the most obstruction loses. Remember that Vitality = Power – Obstruction, Nature's law. The difference between Brother Air's 8½-month fast and a so-called anorexic person is mechanics. Brother Air's body is clean enough to comfortably exist on fruit juice and air, while the anorexic person is running on waste found in the body and will usually break the fast with devastating mucus formers, only to throw it back up. People who are considered to be anorexic are far too filthy to be fasting. Put these people on fruits, green leafy vegetables, some enemas, and we would see some interesting things.

The fundamental theories and philosophies on which medical science is founded are greatly flawed. One day, the sciences may be developed and put to some good use by clean, rational researchers who have knowledge of the mucusless diet and know that pus- and mucus-forming foods are the foundation of human illness. Until then, we must use our own intuitions and knowledge of the system to lead us back to normalcy. We must be patient. The day will come when these so-called doctors and people of science will be coming over here to ask us questions with the same respect and esteem that we are programmed to

---

14. Wikipedia, "B-12 history," accessed 2005, http://en.wikipedia.org /wiki/Vitamin_B12#History.

give them. We are all students attending the colleges of our bodies, authorized and accredited by the Universe. Pay close attention to what your professors say and study long.

Peace, Love, and Breath!

-Professor Spira

Response

Posted on Monday, December 26, 2005 by Wader

Hi Spira!

Your writings make perfect sense. They are absolutely energetic, real, and true. We have been programmed with a certain, inherent fear factor that we must have something outside brought into our bodies for them to be well, as well as being trained into thinking (only partially true in some respects) that disease is caused by an outside source as well. Amazing when simplified. I guess, at times, in transition from their programming, we must be reminded of key points to stay correctly on the path, instead of walking along its outskirts wondrously.

Interesting, the results of the B-12 deficiency testing. I knew we would end up comfortably relying on the perfection of how we were designed to resolve that concern. Thank you so much for that!

"The days of sick, bald creatures in white lab-coats telling us about health are over."

Thank you!! I remember in years past, whenever I was sick, many around me—including close friends—would tell me that I needed to go to the doctor to get checked out. My usual reply to them was why. If a doctor cannot keep themselves from getting sick and/or pass away, how is it that they are going to help me? I would remind them to think back as to how many times they called in for a doctor appointment and were told that their doctor was out "sick"! That is like taking your vehicle in to a mechanic who can never seem to keep their own vehicle running!

Keep up the power and beauty of your work. Have an absolutely wonderful day!

God Bless

-Tim and Samantha Wader

Long-Term Ehretist

Posted by Root on February 25, 2006:

Question: Spira, What can one expect after 10 + years on pure Ehret like Brother Air. You said he's been mucusless for 25-30 years. How much does he eat on a regular basis? Do a handful of grapes satisfy him for a day or two? Does he still have large quantities of food at one sitting? Like a big salad? What is their body composition like?

Spira's Response:

Posted on February 25, 2006 by Professor Spira:

In regard to the different Ehretists I know, it is very interesting to study everybody's results. I am able to see how much of an art form the transition is by seeing the different kinds of results that took place for each individual. The Ehretist who I believe is the strongest physiologically is Brother Air. He has only eaten solid food about 6 months out of the past 3 or 4 years. And he has been consistent with doing long fasts every year. Five years ago he did an entire year of fruit, followed by a 6-month fast the next year, followed by the 8½-month fast last year. He ate for 3 months and then started a fast in September and has been going strong ever since. This is not to mention the years he had achieved mucusless status. At this point, the fasting state is just where he feels the most comfortable and normal. His physiological vigor is relentless; he is constantly on the move. He is a street musician and frequently takes his son out to play. I myself have spent a lot of time playing with him, and it is difficult trying to keep up with the vitality of this 46-year-old who looks like he is in his late 20s. He also sleeps very little during fasting periods, about 15 to 20 minutes every 24 hours. The key to his success has been his masterful ability to stay consistent with the transition and his enemas. His results are merely the conclusion of years of slow and comfortable transition. His 11-year-old son is also a sight to behold. I have never seen a child that emits such joy and light. He is a *Mucusless Diet* baby! He was brought up from birth on the diet, enemas and all. Probably more significant than Brother Air's personal achievements is that of his family unit and how his family revolves around the *Mucusless Diet Healing System* and nothing else. I do not know any other families who can do 5- to 7-day-long family fasts together once a month. Air has taken the diet to a new level and has profound

47

insights into it that nobody else has, because nobody else that we know of has done what he has done in the way that he has done it.

There are others who have also practiced the diet for an extended period of time. Personally, I have always been more interested in what these mucusless diet practitioners have done over the past several decades to sustain the lifestyle than being wowed by their current results. It is easy to marvel at results—such as Brother Air's 8½-month fast—but to really take a hard look at what it took for them to get to where they are physiologically over time is a great education.

These pioneers have definitely picked up where Ehret left off and kept on running. I feel so very privileged to have the opportunity to have unlimited access to their knowledge. For me, it has been essential to study the diet under their tutelage. The refinement that they have brought to practicing the *Mucusless Diet* by living it has been an important part of my modest success in a short time. I look at it like studying music; if I want to become a jazz musician, I must study its origins with Louis Armstrong and New Orleans music. But I also need to check out bebop and what Coltrane was doing in the 1960s. The innovations made since the New Orleans period are essential for study by all jazz musicians who aspire to push the music forward. It is the same thing with rock and roll. Checking out Ehret without studying his successors is like getting into Chuck Berry without checking out Jimi Hendrix. Thus, if one aspires to practice the *Mucusless Diet* today, it is important to understand the contributions and innovations made to it by its long-term practitioners.

Peace, Love, and Breath!

-Professor Spira

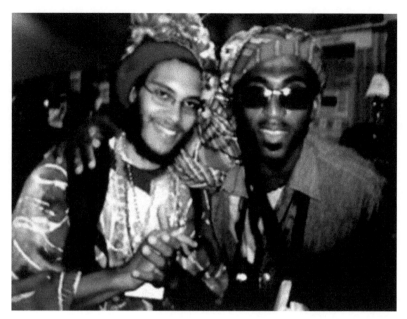

Prof. Spira and Brother Air at PASIC in 2005[15]

---

15. For an extended biography of Brother Air in this book, see page 215.

Do Not Straddle the Barbed-Wire Fence!

Posted on March 25, 2006 by Lachiesa

Question: "Good afternoon, Prof. Spira. I have a couple of questions for you. What advice would you give to an old lady with painful arthritis in her feet? And what advice would you give for a child that has a rare form of leukemia? Right now this child is doing OK with the traditional medicine. However, we all know that it is just a matter of time, and then this disease will eventually kill the kid. Do you think Prof. Ehret's diet would work in these two cases? Thank you so much for your time. I hope to hear from you soon. Keep healthy."

-Lachiesa

Spira's Response:

Posted on March 25 by Professor Spira:

Dear Lachiesa,

For both of the cases that you mentioned, I would recommend the *Mucusless Diet Healing System*. However, if you decide to truly pursue the diet to heal these illnesses, you must not try to straddle the barbed-wire fence that separates Ehret's methods with that of the medical establishment. One of the most dangerous things to do is to stop taking the poisonous medication, half-heartedly practice the diet, and then start taking the drugs again. I know of one person who got a flu shot after she had been practicing the diet for a couple years. The poison from the flu shot was so toxic to her newly cleaned body that she was bedridden for a few days. Dabbling with Ehret while being attached to the erroneous concepts of modern medicine is a recipe for disaster! Once you start traveling down the path of health, you must be steadfast despite the doubts that will arise as you go through painful and frightening eliminations. If you choose to eliminate medicines, then you may need to slowly transition off of them. There are some doctors who will work with you to get off of medicines if you choose to do so. (Disclaimer: this is not medical advice or advice for the treatment of any disease. This is only a sharing of health perspectives and advice on how to navigate certain social situations. You take full responsibility for any decisions that you make related to medicine.)

From the seriousness of both conditions, I would predict that you and the child may have to go through long periods of weakness where lying in bed is about all you can do. You must gather up enough energy to do an enema, but that may be the order of the day: bed, enema, bed, etc. I know that this does not really sound appealing, since our culture is firmly against such selfish acts of personal preservation. The culture is of the opinion that if you are sick or in pain, just take some medicine, eat some food, and get back in the game. The diet demands that you make a choice: you can keep playing the game and be miserable, or you can quit the game and pursue the greatest prize of all—health.

As Arnold Ehret points out, what the medical establishment calls leukemia is nothing more than a condition of constipation where the bloodstream is overflowing with dead white corpuscles. Much care must be taken with the transition for this patient due to the great amount of waste that already exists in the bloodstream. I would recommend really studying the transitional menus and applying them. Proper use of the transitional mucuses such as wheat toast and the vegetable meals will be very important for the beginning of both transitions. Remember that the information in the *Mucusless Diet* book was developed from treating and observing chronically ill patients who were on their so-called "death beds." As always, I recommend trading in the pharmaceutical medicines for boxes of lemons, distilled water, and enema bags. This is the only way to effectively aid the body with its elimination. No medication will ever be able to help the body eliminate pus and mucus. Once you stop putting poisons in and start taking waste out, you will be surprised at how effective your body is as an elimination machine. As long as poisonous medications and mucus are taken into the body, it will appear to stay above water. Once you start taking it away, your physiological addiction to the poison will cry out. The beginning of the road may be a bit rocky, but the reward for your willingness to pursue life will be well worth the work, dedication, and faith.

Health is Wealth!

-Professor Spira

Does Brother Air Eat Avocados and Are They Mucus-Forming?

Posted on March 24, 2006 by Root:

Question: "Spira, I am wondering if your friend Brother Air eats any fat fruits like avocados? Are they mucus-forming?

Spira's Response:

Posted on March 24, 2006 by Professor Spira:

No, Brother Air does not eat avocados because they are terrible mucus formers and are very addictive. Furthermore, it is prudent to just stay away from them unless you crave them, partly for psychological reasons. It is one thing to use them very sparingly at the beginning—if they are craved; but they can become the type of mucus that people feel okay about eating and then get to a point where they never intend to eliminate them from their diet. For both physiological and psychological reasons, the mucus-forming fruits are strongly discouraged, even for the transition. Brother Air always warned me to stay away from avocados because they can become an addictive comfort food. He once asked, "Why would I want to eat a 'fruit' that was like eating French fries?" And he really does not view them as a fruit, but a fatty vegetable. I agree. I prefer to have my fruit eating be mucus/fat-free.

The key area of analysis for avocados is its fat content. Many people do not realize that avocados, nuts, unripe bananas, etc., are potentially mucus-forming if not eliminated quickly enough from the body. However, it must be said that in comparison to other kinds of mucus-forming foods (grains, dairy, meat, etc.), they are far less obstructing. Such items may be used during the transition, but as total mucuslessness is desired, these items would need to be avoided or eliminated completely.

Fatty Fruits and Ehret's Nut Contradiction

Although avocados are not addressed specifically by Ehret—as they did not become a prevalent salad item until the 1950s—Ehret's discussion about nuts can help us to understand the mucus-forming nature of avocados. With that said, the *Mucusless Diet* actually does contradict itself regarding nuts. Ehret writes: "Other kinds of grated nuts, or nut butter, may be served once in a while for this purpose, but are too rich in protein and will produce, if continually used, mucus and

52

uric acid" ("Transition Diet, Part 2" in Ehret, *Mucusless Diet Healing System* [*MDHS*]). In another section he explains, "All nuts are **too rich in protein and fat**, and should be eaten only in winter, and then only sparingly. Nuts should be chewed together with some dried sweet fruits or honey, never with juicy fruits, because water and fat do not mix. With the possible exception of nuts, the above represent about all of the foods which have to be prepared in some manner for eating; in fact they are tasteless unless specially prepared" ("Destructive Diet of Civilization" in *MDHS*).

The contradiction arises when Ehret asserts that "all fruits, raw or cooked, also nuts and green-leaf vegetables are mucus-free" ("Confusion in Dietetics" in *MDHS*). To be clear, nuts are mucus forming. But why was this statement made? There are several explanations for this, but the two main ones are that 1) in comparison with meat, nuts are virtually mucus-free, and 2) that Ehret's editor Fred Hirsch took editorial liberties during the assemblage of the book as we know it and may be responsible for the mishap. Many of these changes or contributions can be easily identified. The greatest example might be in the section, "Vegetarian Recipes," whereby the editor (obviously Hirsch) explains why he added the mucus-lean menus, although Ehret resisted requests to do so.

Ehret ultimately asserted that:

Fats of any kind, including the ordinary butter, are unnatural and therefore should not be eaten. ("Transition Diet" in MDHS)

All fats are acid forming, even those of vegetable origin, and are not used by the body. You will like, crave, and use them only as long as you can still see mucus in the 'magic mirror.' ("Destructive Diet of Civilization" in MDHS)

One of the things that set Ehret apart from allopaths and naturopaths alike is his assertion that the human body does not need, or is unable to use, fats and proteins of any kind. He explains:

High protein foods act as stimulation for a certain time, because they decompose at once in the human body into poison. ("High Protein Foods" in MDHS)

I do have experience eating avocados. When compared to my long stints of living mucus free on grapes, berries, or oranges, avocados are very stimulating and do leave behind slimy residue. I was able to see why many rawists gravitate toward them. I would certainly not eat avocados alone without a salad. I agree with Ehret's recommendation that if fats or protein are craved, a mucus-lean meal may be used. Avocados could be a part of such a meal, but it is best to stay away from them.

In the past, I've conducted observational/boiling experiments similar to Ehret's (see below) on some of these foods to see what kind of residues would be left behind. As observed by Ehret, grapes, dates, etc., leave behind a mucus-free syrup/pap that does not smell bad or become slimy. Yet, I found that masticated nuts or avocados do become slimy, smelly, and leave behind a sticky film. Ehret explains that "the waste from protein and starchy foods is STICKY" ("Magic Mirror" in *MDHS*). This seemed to be consistent with all of the "fatty" fruits I examined. This showed me that such items do not burn away cleanly like grapes, but leave behind obstruction that, if not eliminated, can turn to mucus/uric acid.

Peace, Love, and Breath!

-Prof. Spira

Ehret's Boiling Experiment

Relevant excerpt from *Rational Fasting* regarding Ehret's boiling experiments:

> If potatoes, grain-meal, rice, or the respective meat-materials are boiled long enough, we receive jelly-like slime (mucus) or paste used by bookbinders and carpenters. This mucus substance soon becomes sour, ferments, and forms a bed for fungi, molds, and bacilli. In the process of digestion, which is nothing else but a boiling—a combustion—this slime or paste is being secreted in the same manner, for the blood can use only the ex-digested sugar transformed from starch. The secreted matter, the superfluous product, i.e., this paste or slime, is being completely excreted in the beginning. It is, therefore, easy to understand that in the course of life the intestines and the stomach are gradually being pasted and slimed up to such an extent that this paste of floral and this slime of faunal origin turn into fermentation, clog up the blood vessels and finally decompose the stagnated blood. If figs, dates, or grapes are boiled down thick enough we also

54

receive a pap which, however, does not turn to fermentation and never secretes slime, but which is called syrup. Fruit sugar, the most important thing for the blood, is also sticky, it is true, but is being completely used up by the body as the highest form of fuel, and leaves for excretion only traces of cellulose, which, not being sticky, is promptly excreted and does not ferment. Boiled-down sugar, owing to its resistance against fermentation, is even used for the preservation of food. ("Common Fundamental Cause in the Nature of Diseases" in Ehret, Rational Fasting 1926)

Conversation with Brother Air about Avocados

I talked with Brother Air and he made the following statement regarding avocados:

Peace Brothers and Sisters! I want it to be very clear: avocados are MUCUS-FORMING. There is no debate about this point. And for people who have never tried them, my advice is to stay far away! Avocados are not fruit, but fat. A bad fat, no matter how you combine them! You can't really call it a fruit because fruits help the body eliminate waste, not add to it. Experimenting with avocados is like messing with drugs while playing with fire, don't do it. Even when I ate meat 40 years ago, I was not into avocados. When I started to clean up my diet, I thought to myself, Why would I want to mess with a fruit that is like eating French fries? Why even go there? The purpose of the Mucusless Diet is to help the body eliminate waste, and avocados do not do this.

For some reason, many vegetarians or raw-food eaters gravitate toward the fatty/starchy fruits and vegetables, even if they have never eaten them before. Why is this? It is as if they find these foods for all the wrong reasons. There are thousands of fruits, but the fatty and most stimulating ones become the staples. This is because they are mucus-forming stimulants that get you high.

If you eat or are addicted to them, just know that you need to transition away from them like any other mucus. And then tell us your story. How hard is it to get over an avocado addiction? The avocado should always be marked for elimination and tagged for deletion.

Peace and Respect!

-Brother Air

Habanero Peppers?

Posted on March 26, 2006 by Root

Question: Ok. At the beginning of March 2006 was 1 year on just fruits and veggies. Basically pure mucusless diet. Take 1 week away in Australia (I fell off the Ehret wagon) and I do still eat some avocados. So 51 weeks—almost a year—I can go on like this indefinitely. It's quite easy now. I have done some 3-day just-water fasts. I've done some 10-day just-fruit-juice fasts. I do enemas, colonics, and no chemicals on or in my body. But I know I haven't reached the top yet. I'm waiting for the great feeling you get as Ehret spoke of. Don't get me wrong, I feel good. Also, I still have those boils. So, What now? Do longer fasts? Do you think I have to strip off more layers, so to speak, before I will see more results? Some raw foodists have suggested that I can speed up my elimination with habanero peppers. What do you think?

-Root

Spira's Response:

Posted on March 26, 2006 by Professor Spira

Greetings!

I would definitely avoid habanero peppers and other hot peppers, unless you have an intense craving for them. These types of stimulants produce the illusion that they are eliminating mucus, when in actuality they are just irritating your system and stirring up garbage. You will find that the cleaner your body gets, the more irritating condiments and stimulants such as peppers get. To a clean body, the stench and acidity of hot peppers make them unbearable and useless to eat.

I would be interested to know more about your current eliminations before I would give you a definite recommendation on what to do next. The golf-ball-size boils you spoke of awhile ago usually indicate too hasty of an elimination. If you have been mucusless for the past year, you should really feel some profound changes. But if it is like you said, you feel good but not great, than you may have gone too fast with your transition. How long was your transitional period of cooked, starchless vegetables? Sometimes when you feel that there is a hump you cannot seem to jump over, it is good to take a step back and analyze your practice. You know that you have the physiological prowess and

56

discipline to fast comfortably, and that is wonderful, but is it possible that you need to step back a bit and work on some different layers of mucus in your tissue system, like a runner backing up to get a better and more effective running start?

It is important for the body to go through the various periods of transition continually and systematically over a long time. On the other hand, if you have the desire to engage in a longer fast, go for it. A longer fast will let you actively evaluate your condition. If it is easy and painless, then you know that you are on the right track; but if you start craving the burnt flesh of wild boar eaten by your ancestors thousands of years ago, then you will know what time it is. The key is transitioning the body to the point where it is physiologically impossible to ever fall off of "the wagon," because your body will forbid it. Every time the thought of putting mucus into your body is entertained by your consciousness, you will get that strange repellant feeling that occurs when most people look over the side of a skyscraper. But as long as your body can actually digest mucus-forming foods, there is nothing wrong with using transitional mucuses and cooked, starchless vegetables to move forward.

If you are still craving avocados, I would recommend adding some steamed, starchless vegetables—like broccoli and cabbage—to your salads. When prepared properly, these foods are not too aggressive and are excellent brooms to sweep away the mucus and poisons that your fruit meals have expunged. I think that it would be an excellent shift to trade your avocados for cooked, starchless vegetables. The vegetables won't give you the same high as the avocados, but the weight they provide in your intestines should help with your cravings. I know that you have read some raw-foodist literature and methods; but from the Ehretist standpoint, it is essential not to skip the transitional periods of eating cooked vegetables systematically with fruits. Yes, humans were raw and mucus-free fruitarians before they were vegetable eaters; however, the process to get back to that state includes all areas of the transition. The vegetable phases tend to be downers where you may get a little weak or not feel motivated to do anything. This is okay. We are so used to being stimulated all the time that it takes a great deal of adjustment to learn how to just sit still for a while. For this reason, many people try to stay away from the vegetable periods and hang with eating mostly fruits and fasting—only to have devastating, uncontrolled falls 3 or 4 years down the line. At this point, I would try to get into some serious cooked vegetable periods—even if it is just once a week. If you can do it only once a week and only use it in a medicinal manner, then you know that you have an advanced level of control. If you get deep into the vegetables every day, that is great too. Your body will force you to stop eating cooked and raw vegetables altogether eventually.

How long it will take to gain perfect health cannot be said. We must remember that Ehret was dealing with very sick people who, for the most part, just used his system to keep from certain death. After a few months or a year, they were back to their old eating habits without ever having had the intention of adopting the system as a lifestyle. Ehret was in the process of studying the diet as a lifestyle when he was killed, so we must pick up where he left off. The 3-to-5-year theory that Ehret expounded was not about how long it would take for the body to attain superior health, but how long it would take for your "run of the mill," pathologically sick human being to get clean enough to really start pursuing the diet. And that was for a generation of people who had never been exposed to a Big Mac or ketchup packets. If we are to pursue the diet as a lifestyle, we need to be patient and try to avoid anything that seems like a shortcut. We must pay reparations for the universal laws that we and our ancestors have broken by retracing our steps back to life. Once we have done this, we will return to superior health!

Peace, Love, and Breath!

-Professor Spira

Chapter 3—Consultation with a Mucusless Diet Beginner:

Samantha Claire

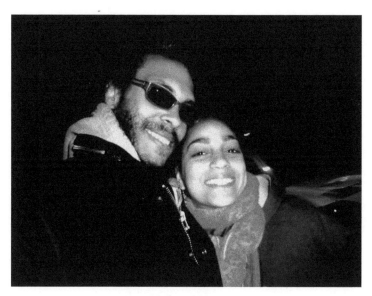

Prof. Spira and Samantha

What Does Spira Mean?

Sent by Samantha Clair on September 19, 2010

Thanks for the videos and the Professor Spira page! I am curious to know why you chose "Spira" as your name.

-Samantha Claire

Spira's Response:

Sent by Prof. Spira on September 20, 2010

Greetings Samantha!

The etymology of the word *spirit* reveals that *spira* or *spiro* means "breath" or "to breathe." Ehret points this out in Chapter V of the *Mucusless Diet Healing System*. He later suggests an interpretation of the concept of "spirit" based on his "air-gas engine" principle of human life. Consequently, he wondered if the idiom "unclean spirits" is really referencing the "bad breath" of a sick or unclean being. As I began to experience the truth of Chapter V, its contents became a profound source of inSPIRAtion for me.

Peace, Love, and Breath!

-Prof. Spira

Confronting Social Challenges in the Beginning

Sent by Samantha Claire on September 20, 2010

How long did it take for you to develop as Spira? I am not even sure if I should phrase it in such a way. Have you become? Developed? Do you turn it on—turn it off? Sooo many questions.

There is a lot of doubt and confusion still going on in my mind about the diet, especially when I am constantly surrounded by people saying, "That's not healthy," and frowning at the idea of the Mucusless Diet, and NO PROTEIN (AHH!) But I am going to try it out for 2 weeks beginning tomorrow (as it is also the first day of Fall, it seems like a good day to begin). Learning takes time. You learn as you do.

Thanks for all of your help and insight. Also, thanks for the essays you've written. The idea of taking enemas is more than intimidating, but I am becoming more and more intrigued as I continue to study Ehret's *Mucusless Diet Healing System.*

I do have some questions to ask you, but I have them written down in my notebook back at the house. The one question I can remember off the top of my head is the "Intestinal Broom." Where in the world could I find all of those herbs? Is there an herb shop you know of in Columbus? Is there something else you would recommend me getting to take as an alternative, or do you recommend the actual intestinal broom blend that Ehret composed himself?

Thanks for all of your guidance and help.

-Sam

Spira's Response:

Sent by Prof. Spira on September 23, 2010

Ehret's Intestinal Broom vs. Enemas

Ehret's Herbal Intestinal Broom is a laxative combination developed particularly for people deathly ill. He would put the laxative in concert with a mucus-free diet, enemas, and periodic fasts to cure individuals who would not have survived otherwise. Then, from the 1930s to the 1980s, Ehret Publishing produced and sold the compound as *Innerclean.* In cases of emergency, it is a good thing to use; however, strategic combinations of dried fruits like prunes and figs followed by juicy fruits can have a similar affect. With that said, for someone who is interested in the diet as a lifestyle, the system including regular enemas renders the herbal remedy somewhat obsolete. I look at the Herbal Broom as something that could be used in emergency situations or in the beginning. The term *Intestinal Broom* can also refer to any vegetable meal where the combination itself has a laxative affect. In practice, fruit and water act as solvents, while vegetables act as an intestinal "broom" to help wipe out what has been loosened.

Enemas and Social Dissonances

The enema component does create an interesting social situation. I notice that for people in the Midwest, it seems crazy or itself unnatural. The fact of the matter is that we have done a devastatingly good job of encumbering our organism with toxic waste and we will have to pay reparations. For me, the greatest technology that is out right now is the enema bag—seriously. So many lives could be saved and changed if people really understood how their bodies worked. In *Bizarro World*, there is such a thing as "routine surgery," where people are actually cut on. Although it may be useful in a small number of instances, using surgery to treat chronic illnesses that are the result of wrong eating is traumatic. A knife is used to cut their body open, obstructions may be redirected or forcibly removed, and the body sewn back up. We are conditioned to find this normal and necessary. But put it up against the enema: a little bit of distilled water and lemon juice in the colon to aid the body in its elimination or be cut apart and sewn back together routinely? I used to take prescription and nonprescription pills every day. I thought it was normal because everyone in my family took many of them. It was almost a rite of passage to have my own prescription. I have not touched any "medication" in over 8 years, and fewer things look crazier to me than to ingest poison when a lot of this "common cold" nonsense could quickly and efficiently be dealt with via fasting, diet, and enemas. I'll take lemon and water over knives and chemicals any day of the week.

That being said, I got into the enemas after beginning to transition. At a certain point, I felt how an enema could really help; and once I began to eliminate the 20-25 pounds of uneliminated waste that I was carrying around inside me, I became a different person to say the least. For beginners, one thing to consider is a colonic. It does not beat or replace consistent lemon enemas, but to attack the immediate waste in the intestines, they can be helpful.

Above, I mentioned the Midwest being behind the times—when I talk with people from Europe, or folks from the West Coast or Florida, they tend to be all over the enemas and colonics. They seem to be much more common in some circles outside of the Midwestern Cave. In fact, many of the so-called stars/celebrities and socio-culturally respected people are actually into colon therapy. Their problem is that many of them may indulge in mucus-forming foods and drugs, only to get with a trainer and colonic operator to take the edge off of their aging process periodically.

It is interesting to me when aspects of these progressive ideas hit the mainstream. Seeing live colonics on Tyra let me know that something is certainly changing. In the 1960s, when the news had video of white firefighters spraying and beating black children, Dick Clark wasn't going to have a colonic demonstration at his American Bandstand.[16] At any rate, as strange as the shift may look, I'm seeing it happen. In the 1980s, could we say that Oprah would have had a live colonic or witness Ronald Regan giving up meat to avoid his tragic demise? Today, Tyra is talking about colonics and Bill Clinton is trying to give up eating meat and dairy. Such things are profound in my eyes because it makes what we do look a little less crazy to the so-called "mainstream." I figure if Bill Clinton can pursue a plant-based diet,[17] then I should at least be able to do year-long fruit fasts and become totally mucus-free. And don't get me started on Mike Tyson attempting to become vegan.

I do understand the enema intimidation. For me, at some point I just decided that I would give it a try for a couple weeks just to see what would happen. Unbelievable transformations began to take place right before my eyes, and I felt and began to look like a different person. At a certain point, I knew that a lot of my friends and peers would try to keep me from pursuing the lifestyle change, and it took great determination and discipline to not feel the urge to tell everyone my business. When people began to question me, I just politely told them the name of the diet and tried to downplay it—like it was just the most normal thing in the world. It did not always keep people from wanting to probe, but anytime that I would share my enthusiasm about the diet

16. For more information about the first live televised colonic on the Tyra Bank's show, visit http://bit.ly/tyra-colonic-crushable.

17. To see Bill Clinton talking about his transition to veganism, see http://youtu.be/aPpcBMwLg2Q.

with HATERS, they would try to rain on my parade. It is certainly one of the great challenges of pioneering the diet in the 2010s. At the early stages, I found inspiration through the sentiments of certain hip-hop ideals, particularly the ones like "I am whatever you say I am," or:

My first name must be He Ain't ish
'Cause every time I'm in a car they be like,
He ain't ish!
I'll be dat, I'll be dat, I'll be dat,
I'll be dat!

That became my attitude. I quit caring what people thought about me and began to embrace the negative ideas thrown my way: "Yup, I'm that crazy dude with the crazy diet and I don't want my piece of the pus (pie), you can have it." I also was driven to viciously study, so that when I was confronted I could defend myself against abuse and know exactly what I'm talking about. But my persistence and efforts to develop ways to discuss this phenomenon have allowed me to now be embraced and respected by many of my peers who no longer feel as threatened. This has enabled me to cohabitate more comfortably. I'm also very grateful to stand on the shoulders of my predecessors who really took the brunt of the social condemnation in the 1970s and 1980s. The reality is that the beginning of the diet is a tender time, and for most, this is a journey that must be taken without the initial support of old friends and family. Without experience and training, trying to explain this diet and lifestyle to others is like trying to explain engineering through interpretive dance or Kabuki Theater. I mention this only because I know how it feels to want to tell everyone about this remarkable information, only to be attacked or have people think that you're trying to preach. Most of those people forget that I did not bring up the diet, but that they asked me a question about why I eat what I eat.

However, it does not take much to be asked questions. Just refuse a food offering and people become very interested in what the deal is. For people who seemingly care little about their own health and diet, they become very interested when you politely refuse some candy or say that you do not eat in restaurants. In fact, I would almost argue that such a reaction is universal, beyond social and ethnic boundaries. At the moment, many people eat and have a concept of what the phenomenon of eating is. When eating is challenged, it creates a dialectical anomaly that forces the creation of a new dialog. But, to what extent are people ready to have such a conversation? How valuable is life, and how great is

64

the desire to forgo the pain and suffering of chronic illness and disease? Who is willing to take the red apple and leave the blue pills alone?

Peace, Love, and Breath!

-Prof. Spira

Navigating Mucus Cravings

Sent by Samantha Claire on September 27, 2010

Spira,

So currently, at this moment, I am craving carbohydrate foods like never before. I want bread, chips and salsa, a spinach wrap, bagels, toast, everything.

I am just confused as to what to eat in such a crisis situation. Should I just eat my baked vegetable with a salad (since I had some homemade applesauce and mashed bananas with a salad for lunch) or should I eat something else as suggested in the book, such as mixed coconut and applesauce? Or nuts? It doesn't seem healthy to just eat nuts and no vegetables.

I am confused, truly.

-Sam

Spira's Response:

Sent by Prof. Spira on September 30, 2010

Greetings Samantha!

The homemade applesauce and mashed bananas sound great! Also, eating a baked vegetable and salad might be the best choice.

As you continue with your transition, you will likely feel old and new food cravings. Your question is one of the best, because having a plan is of the utmost importance so that a binging/relapse period doesn't take you somewhere dangerous and unproductive. Below, I will offer you some menu ideas that have helped me in the past.

First, the starchy items that you crave are the hallmark of a mucus-type (fat)[18] physiology, which is what I am. This is opposed, of course, to the uric acid (lean)[19] type who would likely have uncontrollable cravings for flesh frequently, until the initial cleansing period is completed.

---

18. See page 287 for definition of "mucus-type."

19. See page 290 for definition of "lean-type."

Mucus-Lean Meals to Get Off Meat

One of the mucus-lean[20] meals that helped me kick meat, dairy, and slimier carbs is Hodgson Mills 100-percent-wheat spaghetti. I would make a vegetable tomato sauce by first sautéing some onions/garlic, green peppers, tomatoes, organic Muir Glen sauce, and add slightly steamed broccoli, cabbage, and green zucchini. I would than combine that with the spaghetti and a huge romaine leaf-lettuce salad. If I were still hungry, I would eat a few pieces of well-toasted Ezekiel bread with Willow Creek soy butter (today I would recommend Sahara Valley Hummus with no oil instead, because the soy butter eventually got out of hand and nasty. I currently use no soy butter or hummus, but make my own raw salad dressings in a blender.) A well-baked sweet potato could also be used on hungrier days.

Another mucus-lean meal that helped me get over some humps is beans. I would make the sauté and experiment with different bean combinations. In the beginning, it functioned as "fiber" is supposed to and eliminated fast and well. As I became cleaner, beans became more injurious; but they are a starch that can be used on the transition. I recommend stuff from Whole Foods Grocery, which now has an organic 365 Brand that is as cheap as regular corn-syrup-laden beans. Another mucus-lean choice to consider with care is the Fantastic Nature Burger. It is a combination of various grains that you combine with water, form into patties, cook in a skillet, and then eat combined with a big salad and vegetables. Derivatives of these menus can be used on days of intense craving. Nuts are cool on the transition, but always combine with dried fruit (mainly raisins), which help them eliminate. The idea is to always have a meal that will satisfy, yet be less harmful than what you may actually be craving. As your body becomes cleaner, you will not crave what your body can't handle or should not have.

With all this said, the most important component for anyone truly serious about healing themselves is enemas. Daily colon irrigation is the best way to keep the waste moving, which will help to keep cravings down. Tactfully combining enemas with your food combinations is the key. On a regular day in the beginning of my transition, I would eat a big fruit meal in the afternoon and then do an enema a couple hours before eating my vegetable meal in the evening. Once I was cleaner, I found myself doing enemas first thing in the morning or before bed. After a

---

20. See page 287 for definition of "mucus-lean."

67

while, I began to see the most horrid stuff eliminated—things that I had not recently eaten. When I began to do week-long fasts, I would see 20-inch strands of rotten mucus come out. This level of cleansing would not have occurred that rapidly without knowing how to combine the mucusless diet with fasting and enemas. I encourage those who are skeptical to do enemas consistently for 2 weeks along with the transition and fasting.

Keep in mind, as you begin to cleanse and transition, sometimes you will need to rest. As you go from being stimulated by high-octane mucus-formers to fruits and vegetables, you will probably go through periods of weakness or intense elimination. Part of the American mythocracy[21] is the ideal of John Henry; that is, fasten your boot straps, eat some bacon and eggs, drink some coffee, and get to work!!! Lying down and allowing oneself to be on Nature's Operating Table is usually not a high priority (but if a doctor is cutting off John's arm after fighting for his country, it's okay). I had to allow radical shifts happen to my consciousness as I came to terms with how filthy I truly was/am. For all of the unnatural stimulation that I used in the past (pus/mucus), I have to pay reparations. Sometimes that means focusing on a fast and resting all day.

Letting Go and Surrendering

Brother Air explained to me that I would have to make the choice between letting go and following where the diet led, or trying to make the diet fit into what was my life and have a rough go of things. In other words, I had to choose wholeheartedly to go with the diet or experience unnecessary drama and stress. Once I put the diet in the center of my life, I noticed that the world began to reorder itself around me and my new lifestyle. It became easier to practice the diet, but harder to socialize in the old ways or take part in mucus-inspired occasions. However, once I let go, I seemed to have everything that I needed. I started to focus on what I need instead of what I want. Soon, I was able to meet all of my responsibilities and focus 100 percent on healing. But, when I fought the process and thought that I could have a foot in both worlds, Mother Nature would swiftly punish me in some way. I learned that my health is the most important thing and as long as I put it first, I'll be taken care of.

---

21. See page 287 for the definition of "mythocracy."

When we talk on the phone, I can elaborate further on some of these issues. In the meantime, I can't remember if I sent you all of these or not, but, these are some of Ehret's supplementary writings. The perfect reading material when you're laying down, fasting, blowing your nose, and wondering how much waste is tucked away inside you.

Keep on pushing forward! It will be worth it.

Peace, Love, and Breath!

-Prof. Spira

Readings:

The Definite Cure for Chronic Constipation

Thus Speaketh the Stomach

The Tragedy of Nutrition

Questions about Protein and Water

Sent by Samantha Claire on October 12, 2010

So a question has just run through my mind.

I am still trying to figure out this protein thing, and one of the arguments for it is why eat protein to build protein/maintain protein. But then that makes me wonder about water. If humans are made up of 70 percent water, why consume water? Could the possible answer be because water has oxygen in it, which is vital to our sustainment as living humans? Or is there another reason that we need to drink water as we are mostly water, but we do not need to consume protein even though we are protein.

Do you have any readings on protein? I can say Ehret's short chapter is not enough to read on the matter.

Thanks Spira,

Sam

Spira's Response:

Sent by Prof. Spira on October 12, 2010

Greetings Sam,

I would not consider the statement that you mentioned above to be one of the main arguments against protein, but rather an introductory metaphor for those who have never thought to question such a theory—or who, indeed, do not even know that it is a theory. I'm currently working on a more extensive writing that will be a historical excavation of the protein theory's origins and a critique of its findings. If what Ehret proposes is true, and what I and my colleagues experienced is real, then this information will challenge the basic premise on which Western medical and dietetic science is founded. Scientifically speaking, a seeker of knowledge first considers observable phenomena followed then by their best interpretation and explanation (or conceptualization) of the phenomena. These explanations are intrinsically based upon our current paradigm, that is., systems of thought, reasoning, and belief. If you grow up in a community that performs rain dances to manifest rain, then you will be acculturated to believe in that particular notion of cause and effect, that is, because we dance, it then rains. However, Western

70

reasoning would argue that the weather patterns are not affected by such activities and would endeavor to explain why it rains in what is perceived to be more "scientific" terms. My point is that new information has the potential to totally disrupt what is believed to be unquestionable, for instance, Newtonian physics vs. Einstein's relativity.

Suffice it to say, at first the deconstruction of such hegemonic notions as protein or metabolism may seem arduous, but the fact is that we are the founding mothers and fathers of this new worldview based upon our own experiences—and our own explanations of these experiences. I say this because in 2010, we will be the ones bringing this information to the table. But first, we will have to live it (and then talk about it later). At any rate, a very good introduction to the writing that I'll be preparing on protein is Thomas Kuhn's *Structure of Scientific Revolutions*, which is standard reading in graduate-level studies in the humanities. Read the documents above, respond to the questions found in the Iron and Blood lessons,[22] and get Thomas Kuhn's book from the library. If you would like a more philosophical work to explore that balances Kuhn's, I would suggest Hilton Hotema's *Man's Higher Consciousness* [1962]. We will explore this enigmatic protein theory together.

Peace, Love, and Breath!

-Prof. Spira

P.S. Brother Air might ask you the following: "So you're composed of 70 percent water, huh? Or is it 90 percent? What kind—spring or distilled? What kind of water comes out of your veins when you pierce your flesh? I don't know about you, but I have blood inside my veins." I would probably add, "Although Western reductivism is the modern fad, that is, a close examination of the parts to understand the whole, it can be a very problematic proposition." Brother Air: "Right, you can't see the forest for the trees . . ."

Like many other theories about the human body, the water theory is yet another one that is problematic. Conceptualizing the body in this manner has no real benefit. And drinking water for the sake of drinking water will not alkalize the cells of a body suffering from acidosis.

---

22. See page 227.

Coping with Our Mucus Addiction

Sent by Samantha Claire on October 24, 2010

Dear Professor,

I am an addict, and I cannot get off of my drug. I try. I succeed. Then I fail.

This is a serious issue. People tell me "not to worry," but I feel like I lack self-discipline and control over my own body.

Today I ate a nice combo salad. Then I went to the campus corner store to get cottage cheese, I'm then walking out of the store with ice cream, chocolate covered espresso beans (?), then walked over to get two slices of pizza, a bag of Doritos, a Reeses Crunch Bar (?), and soda.

It's like I can't just have a taste, I have to have it all. I lose so much control.

I have another question to ask. Well, more like a story to tell than a question. This evening, I was hanging out with a friend and talking about the *Mucusless Diet*, and she proceeded to question me about my motives for trying to get rid of mucus. I told her, yet she then persisted to tell me of how mucus lines the organs and without this "moisture" our organs will dry out. Mucus traps and captures foreign agents and then proceeds to eliminate them; so without mucus, our bodies can't trap these foreign agents, and we are more susceptible to disease (blah blah).

Now, I can't just say, "no they don't," but at this moment, that's all I can say, because I haven't even THOUGHT of this argument. I know of us perceiving mucus as a good thing because it is so common in human beings; and because it is found in almost every single person, we believe it is normal (like white blood cells).

My question is, What will happen if our organs are not lined by mucus? Because I am reading online about mucus, but so many damn doctors believe that your lungs will crack if they are not "moistened" by mucus, as it serves to coat and protect our organs,—which I don't believe, but I can't explain WHY I don't believe this. I just know I don't.

Any articles you know that of I can read?

Also, what could be a simple alternative to the ½ stewed prune or dried fruit and ½ cottage cheese combo? I try my hardest to get it down, but cottage cheese is something else.

-Sam

Sent by Samantha Claire on November 1, 2010

Dear Professor,

I have found my way back. It's been about a week, but I have been doing a good job. I plan on staying strong, but I am nervous for Thanksgiving coming up in 3 weeks. And my Grandma, oh Lord. That woman can't remember if I ate or not, so she already asks me 10 times a day if I have eaten; but in addition to that she tries to feed me everything in sight since she forgets.

-Samantha Claire

Spira's Response:

Sent by Prof. Spira on November 2, 2010

The greatest addiction of all time is most definitely mucus-forming foods. Brother Air often says that trying to overcome a mucus addiction makes cocaine and heroin look like getting off of Skittles. The reality is that it will take a long time to overcome the addiction, so do not be hard on yourself. As cravings arise, understand that they are only the expression of poisons that are circulating through your bloodstream. You are not your addiction to mucus, and over time as those poisons dissipate, you will no longer crave the foods that cause harm to your body.

My Baked Banana Surprise is much better than the cottage cheese recipe. Baked Banana Surprise consists of chopped dates and applesauce (brown sugar optional). To bake: take bananas, wrap them unpeeled in aluminum foil, and place on a cookie sheet. Preheat oven to about 415, put in bananas, then bake for about 15-20 minutes. Sweet banana juice should begin to ooze from the side of the foil, which lets you know it's done. Carefully take the foil off, remove the blackened peel, and dump into a bowl. Mix items together and get ready to get high and satisfied. If you do not want to use tinfoil, you can also heat some olive oil in a skillet and slightly cook the bananas to have the same effect. I'm well aware that such a meal would be viewed with scorn among staunch raw foodists, yet such menus could help a lot of people transition in the earlier days of the diet. Further, although it is one of few slightly cooked fruit meals I used, it is basically mucusless. Although it is not the greatest, cooked food is not inherently evil; but cooked or raw mucus-forming foods should be transitioned away from as quickly as possible.

Lymphatic System

The viscous substance identified to be mucus that occurs naturally in the body is not created by, or there because of, eating pus and mucus. Ehret points out:

> First of all, I maintain that in all diseases without exception there exists a tendency by the organism to secrete mucus, and in case of a more advanced stage,—pus (decomposed blood). Of course, every healthy organism must also contain a certain mucus—lymph, a fatty substance of the bowels, etc., of a mucus nature. Every expert will admit this in all catarrhalic cases, from a harmless cold in the nose to inflammation of the lungs and consumption, as well as in epilepsy (attacks showing froth at the mouth—mucus). Where this secretion of mucus does not show freely and openly, as in cases of ear, eye, skin, or stomach trouble; heart diseases, rheumatism, gout, etc.; even in all degrees of insanity, mucus is the main factor of the illness. The natural secretive organs, unable to cope with it longer, the mucus enters the blood causing heat, inflammation, pain, and fever at the respective spot where the vessel-system is probably contracted owing to an overcooling fever (cold), heat, inflammation, pain, fever, etc. (MDHS)

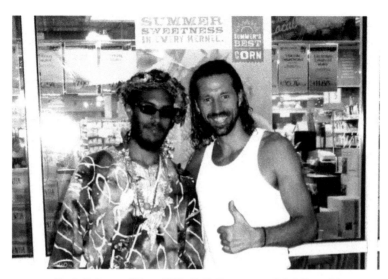

Prof. Spira and Dan "The Life Regenerator" McDonald

Dr. Robert Morse[23] is a great modern-day healer whose work has been substantially influenced by Ehret. I learned about him while watch videos from Dan "The Life Regenerator" McDonald (one of the only online vegan/raw foodists that really speak highly of Ehret's work). He has a clinic in Florida and has practiced naturopathic healing for over 40 years. In this time, he has helped hundreds of thousands of people heal from the most debilitating of illnesses, including paralysis and muscular dystrophy. He uses various levels of fasting, raw-mucusless diet, high-fruit diet, and herbs to heal patients. Ehret is cited as a key influence in the "Acknowledgements" section of his *The Detox Miracle Sourcebook,* and I immediately noticed similarities in the way that he constructs his recommended daily menus. One of the greatest contributions that he has made to the field of naturopathy is his understanding and analysis of the lymphatic system. He points out that the lymph system is a kind of cellular septic tank for the body. But unlike blood, which is pumped by the lungs, nothing pumps lymph fluid. Also, where there is about 3.5 to 5 liters of blood, there is 6 to 10 liters of lymph in the body. In constipated organisms, the lymph system becomes stagnate and does not allow for the elimination of cellular wastes. Yet, fasting and eating astringent fruits can help to get this gigantic lymphatic system moving.

---

23. For more information about Dr. Robert Morse, see www.drmorses herbalhealthclub.com/.

For more on the lymph system, check out some of Morse's YouTube videos entitled The Great Lymphatic System or his *The Detox Miracle Sourcebook*, 2004.

Overall, I think that there needs to be a distinction made between the pus and mucus left in the body, which is derived from uneliminated food substances, and the "lymph" that is naturally found. They are not the same thing, and anyone who thinks that they need to drink milk and eat meat to maintain the moist nature of their cells is out of their mind. Maybe it would be better to call the naturally occurring substance in the body "lymph" and the putrid glue from mucus-forming foods "mucus." Further, the proposition of "white blood" needs to be revisited and reconsidered. Suffice it to say, this is the cutting edge of our physiological studies, and there is much work to be done to better understand this facet of the human body. But such work must be done starting from an Ehretist, or mucusless fruitarian, paradigm to make any further advancement. Such innovations will not be coming from the same consciousness that views meat eating and milk drinking as safe and necessary for human life.

Peace, Love, and Breath!

-Spira

Earthday vs. Birthday

Sent by Samantha Claire on December 16, 2010

Why do you call it Earthday instead of Birthday?

Spira's Response:

Sent by Prof. Spira on December 16, 2010

On the surface, it is meant to be a thoughtful and endearing way to acknowledge someone's day of birth. In the next layer of meaning, there is an underlying connotation that the life of a person is emphasized over that of their birth and death. The word *birth* often presupposes a duality between being born and dying. Etymologically speaking, birth suggests a process of "bearing" or bringing forth life. Within a death culture, the general wisdom is that what is born must die. Rituals often include indulging in poisonous foods and drinks that indeed perpetuate the dying process. Consequently, the meaning of birth and death continue to move further away from the fact of a natural "hue-man" reality. I strive to acknowledge the preeminence of nature and do not take lightly our experience as earth people. If Earth is indeed our Mother, then it is from this life force that we are born. Furthermore, I am convinced that the consciousness of humanity has no beginning or ending. The scientific equivalent of such a notion would be that matter can neither be created nor destroyed, but only changed. If this is true, then what of human consciousness? Thus, I find the semantic insinuation of finality embedded within "birthday" to not be useful.

Peace, Love, and Breath!

-Prof. Spira

Fending off the Naysayers and Haters

Sent by Samantha Claire on January 15, 2011

Sometimes, we must journey before we learn the truth. I am still on the journey but I am trying again. I can picture in my mind the garbage traveling through my body after I eat it. What foods seem like they should be travelling through my blood and through my body? Definitely not french fries.

I have heard too many times, "You can't do that while you live in NYC, it's not possible with all the food." I have heard the same about college. What I am afraid of is the trip to Greece with my family this summer. I recommended to my family that we go to the local markets, buy food, and make our own meals instead of eating out at restaurants, but I was just given "the glare."

I have found, however, that I experience headaches every time I make my salad with cabbage. I think because of the chewing which requires much more muscles and strength than with lettuce, but I don't know how to lessen it. I know Ehret advices to put lemon juice on top of the cabbage for about an hour to soften it, which works, but I am also just not sure of an alternative to so much cabbage.

What do you think?

-Sam

Spira's Response:

Sent by Prof. Spira on January 18, 2011

Greetings Sam!

Ah yes, the naysayers. There will be a lot of those—and many will believe that they are right without any further investigation. Others are terrified by the prospect of the diet and are really just saying, "I can't do it," or "I won't do it in NYC or college." But more frustrating is the "I will talk about something that I do not know anything about with authority" disease. The fact is that most people have not heard anything like what we are talking about; yet instead of saying, "I don't know," they try to find the nearest thing they can relate to it: veganism, macrobiotic, or even fruitarianism, etc., but the *Mucusless Diet* is simply not those things. The implications of V = P - O are unprecedented.

As for "the glare," I hate that. Over the years, I have lived my life in such a way where I rarely have to deal with it anymore. As I think I mentioned before, my approach to such issues has been a bit hardcore. But at the end of the day, I realize that I'm 100 percent responsible for everything that I put into, and eliminate from, my body. Some people may feel offended, threatened, spiteful, or frustrated toward how I've decided to live, but such feelings are reactionary, irrational, and will pass with time. I would rather hurt a few feelings than suffer the consequences of eating materials that I do not need and know will ultimately harm me. One thing that has been interesting to see over the years is how many of the people who gave me such a hard time in the past are now opting to buy fruits and eliminate meat themselves. Deep down, people know that our direction is sound, but to acknowledge it would be to simultaneously recognize that how they live is not righteous. Thus, comments like, "Well if it works for you" sarcastically emerge. It is much harder to rationalize the senseless slaughter of innocent animals and fermentation of their excretions to support masochistic eating habits when we are hanging around talking about fruit diets and fasting.

Avoiding the *Jerry Springer Effect*

It is hard for me to give you specific suggestions for preparing for your trip, since I do not know much about the social dynamics of your family's situation. However, I would probably try to avoid group conversations where it is possible for everyone to gang up on you. I call it the "Jerry Springer Effect."[24] It is much easier for people to rationalize the normalcy of their addiction if they maintain solidarity. I've warned other friends not to enter "Mucusland" territory without backup. Most Crips [famous gang] wouldn't confront a gang of Bloods [rival gang] without their boys having their back. The US military doesn't send one solder into war without their platoons and regiments. That being said, calm, rational discussions with individual family members away from food and drink may be the best way to let people know that you are serious about what you are trying to do. Although you refuse to compromise about what you put into your body, you may reassure them that your actions are in no way meant to be disrespectful.

---

24. See page 286 for definition of "Jerry Springer Effect."

(To strengthen these skills, I used to watch the adversarial white folks vs. Malcolm X interviews, for example: http://youtu.be /ENHP89mLWOY)

. Thus, you mean not to impose on them with your dietary beliefs. An apt compromise would be that you ensure that you can get the fruits and vegetables that you need without forcing them to eat like you. It seems that you got the glare because your suggestion included that everyone go shopping with you and eat homemade meals. Such a proposition could be perceived to be imposing. However, you are well within your right to assert that you will be buying your food from local markets and maintaining your own dietary regimen. Being steadfast, yet non-imposing, should eventually earn a newfound respect where people go out of their way to help you and give you what you need. For the longest time, people tried to offer me vegetarian foods or try to invite me to vegan restaurants as a thoughtful gesture, yet I still kindly declined. After a while, people started asking me what I would accept, which sometimes resulted in people buying me boxes of lemons, apples, and oranges. Although this approach may initially create a certain kind of isolation, over time it becomes accepted and respected by those around you. My family knows that I'm not going to be hanging around on "Thankskilling" or Halloween, but I'm able celebrate life with them in other ways that are not predicated on eating.

Preparing to Travel

With Greece, I would do as much research as possible about where you are staying. Check out Google Earth for a lay of the land and general Google searches to learn of nearby markets, e.g.:

http://www.greecefoods.com/farmers-markets/index.htm.

I would also find out as much as I could about the nearby general grocery stores. Once you learn more about what you have access to, you will be better able to transition and prepare for your trip. The more knowledgeable you are about the specifics the better. If there are transitional items that you use a lot now, but will be hard to obtain on your trip, try to find something else to use or move on from the addiction. Although it might not be necessary for Greece, it is also good to make sure that there are no policies or laws that try to force you into getting shots. There are many websites and books on how to navigate such reprehensible policies. I've not fully reviewed it yet, but this website and book looks like a good place to start: How To Legally Say "NO" To

All Vaccines (visit www.bit.ly/say-no-to-vaccines) and Saying No to Vaccines: A Resource Guide for All Ages, by Dr. Sherri Tenpenny (visit http://bit.ly/no-to-vaccines-tenpenny).

Firm vs. Soft Green, Leafy Vegetables

Regarding cabbage, I actually usually advocate a softer raw salad of green/red/romaine leaf lettuce and spinach, combined with finely cut carrots and celery. Cucumbers, green peppers, etc. may also make nice additions, but the primary foundation is the leaf lettuce. This is a bit different from Ehret, who places a greater emphasis on the bulkier raw ingredients like cabbage, with lettuce being used for taste. I prefer lightly steamed cabbage either put on top of the salad or eaten separately with tomato sauce. In the end, it is all about elimination. The folks that Ehret wrote for could use a bulkier cabbage effect; whereas I think that our physiologies are able to go further with softer leafs. Also, from a historical perspective, cabbage is a very practical leafy vegetable. It lasts a long time without refrigeration. Many people presumably did not have the same kind of access that we have to fresh leaf lettuce and greens every day. For me, a perfect raw leaf meal consists of eating several leaves directly from a head of lettuce with a carrot or piece of celery. Over the years, I have transitioned away from elaborate salads toward ones that are as simple as possible.

French Fries and White Potatoes

French fries certainly contribute to garbage circulation in the body. I think I ate my last french fry when I learned that many restaurants use the same chemicals to freeze and preserve them as they do to preserve dead bodies and make drugs like PCP. Either way you look at it, it's about preserving dead bodies. The white potato is definitely on the *"do not consider eating'* list. It is always better to opt for sweet potato treats. Baked is best, but sweet potato chips or fries may help get you past a white potato chip or fry craving. Personally, I tried to stay away from making my own peanut-oil sweet potato fries because I knew I would become too addicted to them. However, such an option is much better than any kind of white potato madness.

Fall Options (Mucus-Lean Menus)

One thing that you want to do is develop what I call "fall" options for the times when you feel like you're falling off the wagon. Consider what you are craving and find a better option. Usually the better option is not something that you will want to eat forever, but it may be a lot better than the crazy craving. This is where a conscientious usage of soy-based vegetarian products may come in handy. I used starch meals consisting of various kinds of beans and corn chips in the early days to overcome comparatively worse cravings. However, I always surrounded such meals with a lot of leaves and vegetables. Combined with consistent enemas, I always eventually leave the worse cravings behind, permanently.

Peace, Love, and Breath!

-Prof. Spira

Sent by Samantha Claire on January 19, 2011

You truly are amazing. You have done nothing but given all you can to help me and I truly appreciate this.

-Samantha Claire

Is it Okay to Fast?

Sent by Samantha Claire on February 15, 2011

Question:

Is it okay to do a 1-day fast at this ~~f~~ of my transition? I have been on it for like 5 weeks now, I have ~~dairy~~ or meat, but an occasional slip up that was never really too ba~~d~~

I am just wondering how you would "break" a 1-day fast? Do I wait till the next day or do I wait until later in the first day?

Spira's Response:

Sent by Prof. Spira on February 16, 2011

Greetings!

Cooked vs. Fresh Juices

It should be okay to do a 1- or 2-day fast. Are you considering a dry fast or juice? As recommended by Ehret, I think a juice fast with your favorite juice would be good. When I first started the diet, I did a lot of Welch's 100 percent grape juice fasts and then moved to the Dole (not from concentrate) pineapple juice in a can. As I learned how to make fresh juice, I opted for fresh over *cooked* store-bought juice more and more. Today, cooked juices in a can or carton taste horrible to me. Now, I always try to drink freshly squeezed juices whenever possible.

Breaking the Fast

Your question about breaking the fast is very good. Breaking a fast properly is of the utmost importance.

<u>Rule number 1</u>—Do not break a fast with any mucus-forming foods.

In fact, try to eat mucusless for several days after breaking it. What you do not want to have happen is to lose control if you start craving a bunch of mucus. With breaking the fast, you can either do it with a fruit meal or a vegetable meal. The fruit meal is more aggressive, and if you are not clean enough, you could crave mucus. A very laxative vegetable meal or salad can be beneficial. The key is to eat foods that create a laxative effect and travel through the intestines fast and efficiently.

<u>Rule number 2</u>—Do consistent enemas.

In light of the above, one of the most important things in all this is to be doing enemas to keep the waste moving. Of course I advocate and practice daily lemon enemas; it is particularly important when fasting. When you fast, the waste begins to eliminate. However, in the constipated condition that we are in, our bodies are unable to fully eliminate the filth. A well-timed enema can do much to eliminate the 15-20 pounds of caked-on waste in the intestines. Even people who have regularly fasted and eaten plant-based for years are dumbfounded by the amount of waste that they were harboring when they start to do enemas. Alas, the enema was first developed in Egypt—as the story goes—when a Pharaoh became sick and witnessed some birds that shoot water into their colons with their long beaks. He requested a tube be made from cane and endeavored to irrigate his colon. The practice became a regular part of hygiene or medical practice for many peoples, including folks from the equatorial forests in central Africa, the Mayans and Amerindians, tenth century Sung Dynasty, and Hippocrates (the so-called founding father of Western medicine, etc.). Check out this short history: http://www.enemahistory.com/.

I emphasize this because I know that it is a bit taboo from our standard American frame of reference. I resisted at first, like many people; but when I started to do them, I transformed my life quickly. Within weeks, I started to see long thick strands of tar-like mucoid plaque eliminate from my bowels. Not to mention the terrible stench. Death smells bad, and I had plenty of death just sitting in my intestines. The key was that I used the enemas as part of the system. When I fasted, instead of running on my accumulated waste, my organism was able to get cleaner in a shorter amount of time.

In sum, I think that you are certainly ready to do some fasting. Just be sure to surround yourself in as calm of an environment as you can. When you fast, you are on Mother Nature's operating table and the healing takes time. But it is well worth the effort.

Peace, Love, and Breath!

-Prof. Spira

Sent by Samantha Claire on February 16, 2011

So I made it through my first 1-day fast. I drank delicious apple juice throughout the day and I am still awake. Who needs coffee?

My question is, which vegetables serve as the best laxatives after I break the fast? I have done a little reading and I saw that leafy greens are good, as well as carrots and broccoli. I just prepared my specialty salad of onions (mmmm), dark lettuce, stewed cabbage, and carrots. Do you think that is good enough? I hope so; it took me 20 minutes to prepare it.

Also, is it too early to begin trying out enemas? Or should I wait a little longer? Oh, and if you recommend exploring it at this time of my journey, what should I get? It's like shopping for my first bra all over again. I just don't know—but want to know so much.

Thanks for your guidance. I sincerely appreciate it.

-Sam

Sent by Prof. Spira on February 17, 2011

Greetings Sam!

Your vegetable combination salad sounds good to me. As you eat, take note of how it makes you feel and how quickly it eliminates from your system. Over time, you will be able to tweak these meals so that they can be as laxative as possible for your own body. Your selections are certainly a good place to start.

Never Too Early to Begin Enemas

In my opinion, it is never too early to begin the enemas. There are so many illnesses that could be dealt with by simply cleaning out the putrid filth that lies within the colon/intestines. Ehret points out that the "no breakfast plan" alone can cure many acute illnesses, and I would add that when combined with enemas, an even greater transformation can occur. Many of the so-called "medical professionals" who are against enemas base their assertions on data from constipated pus- and mucus-eaters—not people who have been doing enemas every day for many years. They try to claim that enemas will constipate you or cause you to depend upon them for elimination. This has not been the case for me at all. I have plenty of eliminations without enemas. The constipation myth comes from doctors shooting a little water into a terribly constipated person (who is presumably not eating mucusless foods) for a couple of days and expecting something to happen. The fact of the matter is they do not know anything about combining enemas—as daily hygiene—with the mucusless diet.

Where to Get Enema Supplies

What you want to get is an enema/douche combination package. These are sold mostly at old-school medical supply stores. See if there are any such stores in Delaware. There is a spot on High Street in Columbus where I get mine. Also, most CVS stores also carry enema bags in the feminine hygiene section. If you cannot find one and would like for me to grab one for you let me know. Details about doing the enema may be found in my "What Do We Need to Eat" essay.[25] Also, never use Fleet enemas, and don't get a little bulb enema meant for babies (like I first did). The only liquids that really should be used are warm, distilled water and lemon juice.

Doing Enemas in a House Filled With People

Given that enemas are still considered taboo in this part of the country, if you feel a bit self-conscious about your housemates, you can always turn on the shower while you do it. Crank up the music, light some incense, and you're good. For my first 2 years of the diet, I did enemas in a lockable public bathroom in the dorms. One bathroom was near a pool table and another in the TV room. Some people would give me funny looks for going into the bathroom with a big duffel bag for 30 min, but it didn't bother me. Health is much more important to me than worrying about what these folks think. I juiced my lemons in my dorm room, heated my water in the kitchen up the hall, filled my bag, put everything in a black Adidas bag, and went downstairs. And when I would spend the night with my family—or anywhere—I just did what I needed to do. I usually explained my case to people early on and then tended to my business. Wherever I go, my distilled water, lemons, and juicer go with me.

After having met your family, my initial sense is that you may have to take a little different approach than I did with mine. The famous saying goes, "A prophet is not without honor, except in their own

---

25. See page 9.

village," and I knew that I was going to have little success explaining certain things. I did buy Ehret's books for all of my closest family and friends, and gave them some informative literature. But, my outlet for the message became the lifestyle itself as expressed through my art/music. For the most part, I was just left alone by my family to do what I needed to do. In your case, it seems like you might need to come to the table more boldly a bit earlier—with pictures of intestinal grime and pathology—to explain why you do what you are doing.

Let me know if you have any further questions.

Peace, Love, and Breath!

-Prof. Spira

Sent by Samantha Claire on February 22, 2011

Spira,

Is there a point where you just feel down about 60 percent of the time? Is this my withdrawal coming out?

-Sam

Sent by Prof. Spira on February 22, 2011

Dealing with Mood Swings

On one hand, you will undoubtedly begin to "come down" and at times feel bad and depressed. It is a sensitive time when you need to surround yourself with positive people and atmospheres while eliminating negative ones. Restricting the stimulating foods that you previously ate/drank/smoked/etc. can make you feel down. Very low! This is where it is interesting to examine the potential of the body versus your mind and emotions. I found that my body is able to advance much faster than my mind, thus I feel that I need to work harder on mentally preparing than the physical practice itself. The reality shift that occurs as a result of making these changes results in a true rebirth. With that said, Vitality = Power - Obstruction; if you have yet to irrigate your colon, you are not going to feel very good. Through your diet, you are loosening up decades of waste, but our condition does not allow for us to eliminate it as efficiently as need be. At this point, I think that there is much work to be done in the bathroom.

-Prof. Spira

Shaking the Mucus Down

Sent by Samantha Claire on March 1, 2011

Hey, I got your missed call. I've been studying. Well, I thought I was supposed to be, but didn't quite and now I'm still awake. But on the bright side, I did my first enema.

Peace.

Spira's Response:

Sent by Prof. Spira on March 1, 2011

A very bright side, indeed. Baptism!!! (And no little chicks were harmed, LOL [reference to the famous PETA slaughterhouse video where young chicks are tortured]).

Sent by Samantha Claire on March 28, 2011

I know we haven't spoken in a while, but I wanted to share some great news.

I woke up this morning as my nose was leaking uncontrollably with mucus. I don't have a cold or the sniffles now that it has been an hour. It was my elimination! Ahhh. How cool. I'm still continuing on. It has almost been 3 months (11 weeks).

It's even to the point where I'm craving salads. I am still craving other stuff but hey, if I'm sitting down and having an itch for some greenery, I think I'm well on my way.

-Sam

Sent by Prof. Spira on March 28, 2011

Yeah! Let that old stuff drain on out! I'm glad to hear that it's starting to loosen up and move. It's also great that you're starting to really crave salads. Keep up the good work!

Sent by Samantha Claire on March 30, 2011

Did you ever feel like your nose was runny but your nasal area was dried out? It's such a strange feeling I am experiencing right now. Two days ago, I felt fatigued like hell. Yesterday I was nauseous, and today I feel tired, yet runny. How bizarre.

-Sam

Sent by Prof. Spira on March 30, 2011

Samantha,

I think the medical profession calls that post-nasal drip. The allergy medication that I used to be on caused me to go through that on a daily basis for many years. However, now that you are eliminating, you should see mucus and pus try to leave the body anywhere it can. Increased eye crust, stinky ear wax, increased dead skin cells (on feet), etc. The mucus that you are eliminating now is probably extremely salty. This salt dries out your nasal cavity. With post-nasal drip, salty mucus drips down the back of your throat instead of coming out through your nose. It is certainly one of the more unpleasant kinds of elimination.

Developing a Mucusless Lifestyle

From early on, I learned to use such eliminations to my advantage. Whenever I started to go through that level of elimination, I first accepted my condition and immediately began to fast and meditate. As I focused on my breath I would think about the laws of cause and effect. Although I experienced pleasure years ago while eating dead animals, I now feel the pain while it eliminates. How many times did I pop a pill to suppress elimination? By thinking deeply, I was able gain an understanding of my condition that enabled me to push forward with courage. Fasting combined with enemas, meditation, *Coltrane Live in Japan* [music recording], and rest became my new habits. I avoided negative external diversions and focused on my fasting and breath. The periods of weakness can be frightening, but I understood that I was only going through what I would have inevitably experienced in old age or beyond. Better to go through it with a more youthful body. If I needed to miss class, I did so and gave my professors a copy of the *Mucusless Diet Healing System* while affirming that I do not go to doctors for such matters.

Elimination is certainly bizarre, but it is actually bringing us back to normality. Pill popping and animal eating are completely bizarre and against the laws of nature. In a world where abnormality defines normality, you are looked at with scorn when you fast and irrigate your colon. But, this is about a real struggle to survive. Our ancestors freed themselves from unimaginable hardships, but the fight for liberation is not over yet. Physiological liberation is the struggle of all struggles.

Really, it is a blessing to go through these eliminations. Keep on pushing!

Peace, Love, and Breath!

-Prof. Spira

Sent by Samantha Claire on March 30, 2011

This is mind blowing!

It's interesting, because I feel as if I am constantly dehydrated, tired, and have a headache. But I am not afraid. I am excited! That morning I woke up and immediately did an enema. I was so happy that I may have told too many people that I woke up in a pool of mucus.

But what is also weird is that I feel like I can breathe so much better. A new air passage that has been blocked has now been cleared and breathing feels so good. For almost a year I have been trying to be conscious of my breath without altering it to what I want it to be because I often felt as if I never breathed deeply but took short little breaths. And now that the drip has taken place, I can breathe! How magnificent.

-Sam

Sent by Prof. Spira on March 31, 2011

Sam,

Those are the kind of details that you have to experience to believe and understand the truth. You are beginning to enter into an area that most people have not yet been exposed to. In the annals of history there are very few texts that explicitly talk about the physical elements involved with this kind of elimination. Your story reminds me of when I first started breathing better after a great elimination. It really was the closest thing to a literal "rebirth!"

-Spira

More Cravings

Sent by Samantha Claire on April 3, 2011

BTW,

My cravings are worse than ever. I want fried chicken and snacks, snacks, snacks, and bacon. Geeeez.

Spira's Response:

Sent by Prof. Spira on April 4, 2011

Sam,

Yup, it's crave time. You have experienced some of the fruits of your labor and see the potential (e.g., your improved breathing), but now the hard work really begins. Physiological karma is a monster. When you have those cravings, what do you usually eat or do? Have you found a transitional meal that calms the cravings? Or, if you are like me, you do an enema when the really bad cravings come.

The transition of the seasons agitates such eliminations even more (think about the effect of cold-to-warm temperatures on the body). Before the diet, I seemed to eat (and act) my worst in the Fall and Spring, especially Spring. I've had to keep that in mind as I develop strategies to overcome certain challenges during those months.

Lately, I've been going through a craving for 100-percent-wheat crackers and toasted wheat flatbread. This is an improvement from my addiction to corn chips in the past, but I must strive to get over this hump soon. I fasted for a few days last week, and that is certainly where I'd rather be at. But there are a couple more goals that I aim to complete before earning another long fast.

Stay away from that old fried chicken and bacon, LOL! Keep on pushin'.

-Spira

Sent by Prof. Spira on December 8, 2011

You get a special sneak peek. I have a lot a material that are about to be released into the time capsule we call the "the internet."

Immortality Pipeline Teaser: Talking about the Mucusless Community and Fasting (visit www.bit.ly/mucusless-community-video)

Join Prof. Spira, Brother Air, and Baby Babaji as they talk about Arnold Ehret and their experiences practicing the *Mucusless Diet Healing System.*

Immortality Pipeline: Practicing the Mucusless Diet during Pregnancy 2/13/08 (visit www.bit.ly/mucusless-diet-pregnancy)

In this excerpt, Prof. Spira, Brother Air, and Baby Babaji talk with a pregnant practitioner of the *Mucusless Diet* about her five vegan pregnancies and raising children Mucusless.

Sent by Samantha Claire on December 8, 2011

YES!

Elimination Mode

Sent by Samantha Claire on December 10, 2011

Spira!

Since I am currently in elimination mode, I have not been in the mood to talk to anyone on the phone. I have just been lying in my bed and "hawking up loogies" right into my spit cup.

So when I am back in full gear, I will give you a call.

I do have a question. Since I am in elimination mode, I have been doing enemas, but I feel like I have a whole bunch of mucus stuck in my nasal cavity and the back of my throat, which is being eliminated quite slowly. Do you have a special remedy for loosening that up?

Also, I have not wanted to drink or eat anything, so I have not had even a sip of water (except I did make some warm apple cider which is not doing my stomach well, and my body is still really hot even though I drank it over and hour ago). I am taking this as a sign to not drink anything if my body says "no."

Or am I missing something?

This is my first elimination since last April. I have not had a "cold" or anything this entire fall and thought I was doing well; but now in December, here it is. Mucus loosening up! Mucus in my blood, circulating.

Mannn—the crazy cravings I've been getting. I was walking down the street and all of a sudden I was like, "scallion cream cheese!" And "peanut butter jelly sandwich." RANDOMLY!

Any thoughts?

-Sam

Spira's Response:

Sent by Prof. Spira on December 10, 2011

Greetings Sam!

I'm glad to hear that you are in *elimination mode*! I'm right with you. I know that it is so very uncomfortable, but just let it drain. As the gallons of mucus start to pour out, you begin to learn what cannot be explained in any book or understood through a conversation or lecture. When you think about it, this may be your first or second drug-free, food-free elimination. You are now coming down and sobering up from years of eating stimulating foods and suppressing eliminations with poisons. Now you will come to know what those foods and drugs actually did to your body. When I experienced my first big elimination after beginning the diet, I went through multiple boxes of tissues every day for a while. I began walking around CCM with a box of tissues in one hand and a spit bag in the other.

If you don't feel like eating or drinking, then don't (I wouldn't). However, bear in mind that you do not want to fall into an uncontrollable binge (if you can avoid it). When I was learning how to fast, I would keep lettuce, celery, carrots, and spinach in the fridge (for the first week at least). I would be going along good and then hit some crazy craving, as you are experiencing, and then fill my stomach with a combination salad/GI broom. After this, I would sometimes fall from grace and find myself at the store or in the kitchen making some very strange concoctions; but don't let such things ever make you feel guilty. Keep doing the enemas, blowing your nose, hawking loogies, and going forward. You can always return to the fast.

With accumulations of thick mucus in the nasal cavity and throat, I break out the warm lemon water. Juice a couple lemons and heat up some water. I gargle a mouthful and spit it out. Then gargle and swallow. I would do this a couple hours before enemas, or after them. For me, lemons have always been an omnipotent loosener. Then I would juice fast, usually on either orange or grape juice. If the elimination became too aggressive, I would drink warm vegetable broth. (It was an organic store bought brand. I tried making Ehret's veggie broth a couple times and always was unable to resist eating the vegetables).

Overall, rest as much as you can. Although your body may become weak, your mind should become clear. I would often lie down and meditate on my past food addictions and try to wrap my mind around the depth of this path.

I hope this helps. If you have any more questions, feel free to ask.

Peace, Love, and Breath!

-Spira

Another video to check out:

What It Takes to Practice a Mucusless Lifestyle on Immortality Pipeline, 8-27-06 (visit www.bit.ly/mucusless-diet-practice)

Daktehu joins Prof. Spira, Brother Air, and Baby Babaji on the Immortality Pipeline to talk about dealing with friend and family relationships while practicing the *Mucusless Diet*.

Life Challenges on the Diet

Sent by Samantha Claire on December 13, 2011

Hello Brother Spira,

Today is Day 7 of my fast. I have had a couple of pieces of fruit every day to refresh my taste buds (and BOY—organic Valencia oranges are the BOMB!). I currently am feeling intense mood swings and lethargy, but this usually happens to me by the end of the day. When I first wake up, I feel great. Although I do not follow her dietary guidelines to the T, in Queen Afua's *Heal Thyself for Health and Regeneration* book, she mentions that by the second week of the fast we feel more energetic and less angry. Keeping in mind that every person is different, and I did not consciously begin this fast, I will not be let down if this is not the case. However I would LOVE to have an upswing in mood.

What is your theory behind the mood swings?

I know when I have eaten meat since I have begun my sojourn, I notice an immense shift in my mood. Now, I know people tend to get quite irritable when they have not had food in a while, but I believe that as the mucus that is loosening up (all of these toxins I have ingested within over 21.5 years) and is back in my circulation, my mood is being shifted left and right.

I said some terrible things to my sister about a half hour ago, but I am living with the most unsupportive people (except my mother, surprisingly, perhaps because she is a Christian and Christians fast, although she has never fasted because that's a thing Man has created). My dad said he is over this "anorexia mess," and my sister said I am malnourished, and I have replied with, "Leave me alone and enjoy your cancer." Now, that was not the most positive thing for me to say to my loved ones; however, they honestly made me so mad that I never wanted to see them again. I feel like I can't live with them; however, I can't *not* live with them. It's way too expensive in NYC, and I am tied down to my job right now. (I can't leave my kids after just beginning violin lessons with them!)

Everyone always has to tell people what to do. EVERYONE. Especially if you are doing something soooo far off from the majority of the S.A.D. People say, "You NEED to eat." Ugh!

My dad has a patient who is really awesome, but she is very receptive to the different dimensions of the Earth and Universe (such as she could physically feel the arrival of the earthquake we had in August, to the point where she felt herself shoot out of her body. Most people consider her crazy; I believe she is a gift). She, however, went on about how my Chi was off and brought me raw oatmeal because I need to eat. And I'm like, "If I were to break my fast on this raw oatmeal, I COULD DIE!!!" People have no idea, but think they know the truth. At the same time, who am I?

Also, my question is, that supposed "hunger" feeling we get when our stomach grumbles is just the mucus loosening from our stomach? Usually after that sensation I feel dizzy and nauseous.

Let me know your thoughts on all my scattered thoughts as I am still bedridden. My dad is having his second hip surgery tomorrow, so I don't want to cough all around him. He's like, "Your GERMS!"

Also, what do you think about the "contagiousness" of eliminations? When people have colds, they are contagious. Or how is it that when one person gets a cold, a whole community of people also gets it at the same time? Isn't a cold just an elimination? Do you have an idea as to how this works?

Much love,

Sam

Spira's Response:

Sent by Prof. Spira on December 15, 2011

Greetings Sam!

Well done on 7 days! It sounds like you are really starting to get deep into your elimination. The mood swings are definitely a big part of the detoxification process in the beginning. It is hard to say how long it will persist, but know that it will eventually end. Although the lows can feel like they will go on forever and the highs are euphoric, as the poisons leave you will balance out. I know that you enjoyed a little cannabis in the past, and you can definitely look for those eliminations to be intense and strange. The important thing is to stay focused on the fast and your elimination, no matter how you feel.

I'm sorry to hear about the family. As you get deeper into the diet, it could get worse before it gets better. To balance out my "worldly" interactions and emotional eliminations, I've studied and practiced various forms of meditation and contemplation. If you are interested, I could tell you more about that part of my journey. But overall, sitting calmly and focusing on your breath as long as you can is a great start. When you "balance out," I would not expect to feel like your "old self," but a new you. Be patient with the people around you, as they will need time to get to know the new you.

Buddha's Broken Fast

The raw oatmeal is interesting. It was said that after fasting and meditating under a tree for 7 years, Buddha broke his fast with rice offered to him by a concerned woman. After eating the rice, the enlightened beings (I suspect breathaireans) he was talking with left him. There are strong forces at work that will do everything in their power to keep you in the world of pus-eating. Contemplation, meditation, and getting deeper into the study of your own physiology can help you to move toward a state of calmness in the midst of some of the most bizarre human reactions you will ever see.

People certainly have no idea. Yet, there is a time for all things. There will be great need for you to share your knowledge with others, but now you must heal and free yourself. Let go of anything that feels like "wanting to change other people," and focus on your own "I am-ness." Have compassion for others, since you know they do not understand; but release yourself from wanting to explain what you are doing. If you stay steadfast, your time with the microphone will come, and you will be met with love and respect for sharing your knowledge.

Hunger Pangs

Hunger pangs are waste and acids secreted from your stomach and intestines, and not indicative of real hunger. Your body is expecting to work on food from years of regular eating, so acids are secreted. It is said that real hunger is in the throat, although I've never gone that far and it's not advisable to do so. I usually break a fast when I feel that there is a lot of loosened waste in my system that is not coming out in my colon or through my kidneys. One of the reasons I am so adamant about enemas, particularly the lemon, is to combat the unimaginable toxicity in the GI track. As that stuff is brought to the surface, it is very important to get it out as soon as possible. Depending on what is recirculating, the dizziness is a nasty side effect. Yet, if you ever consumed any pharmaceutical medication in your life, you can expect to experience every one of those side effects listed on the warning label as it leaves the body. Dizziness is often a sign of such poisons leaving. If it persists for a longer time, your body could be repairing some of your weaker glands.

Concept of Contagious Disease

Our concept of "contagions" is like a carryover from medieval times. Then, disease was blamed on an evil spirit that possessed the body and could infect others nearby. The theory of bacteria and viruses causing illness has taken the place of the "evil spirit," yet it is fundamentally the same in that it has to do with an external agent entering the body. Then, according to science fiction, these germs can be passed from host to host and cause sickness. First, in order to get sick you must have a nice amount of waste in the body. If there is no waste, then bacteria and viruses have nothing to munch on and cannot affect you. If an external agent does start messing with you, then it can help you eliminate by feeding on the waste you don't need. Your body reacts with flu-like symptoms, which is a great thing. There are many explanations for the phenomenon of multiple people getting sick together. First, the mind and symbiotic nature of humans is power. Since it is thought that germs are contagious, the minds and bodies of people can trigger elimination. But if there is no waste, such triggers cannot happen. In extreme cases like the European plague that almost wiped out everyone in Europe and current African plagues (Ebola, etc.), the combination of a toxic body with an ancient virus is too much. With knowledge of the *Mucusless Diet* and access to fresh fruits and vegetables, major plagues could be halted immediately. Imagine what you are unearthing and unleashing back into the earth with your elimination. Some the toxic waste may be ancient and very hungry for a new host. Woe to those who may encounter our ancient eliminations.

As more people begin to cleanse on this level, it will be much harder for others to survive without following suit. Mother Nature does not play any games and will eliminate the waste. Get the waste out of yourself and get out of the way because it is not going to be pretty.

There is more that can be said on the subject, but I'll leave it there for now. Keep on plugging along. Listen to your body and let the naysayers to their grumbling. You have the key, go with it!

Peace, Love, and Breath!

-Spira

Check out this wonderful talk given by my friend Brother Air:

Brother Air's Keynote Address at the Booker T. Washington Holistic Health Fair (visit www.bit.ly/brother-air-talk)

Brother Air shares his experiences practicing Prof. Arnold Ehret's *Mucusless Diet Healing System* at the Booker T. Washington Holistic Health Fair.

Fast-Breaking Techniques

Sent by Samantha Claire on December 15, 2011

Thank you my brother!

So thinking about breaking the fast, what do you recommend to break a fast with? I remember reading a paper you wrote about fasting and how to not break it with mucus-producing foods and breaking it with fruit can lead to more intense craving. What do you usually do? How long does it take for your body to get back in to the swing of eating full meals? Does it take you several days to get back?

Spira's Response:

Sent by Prof. Spira on December 16, 2011

Fast-breaking technique depends upon your condition. In the early days, I treated myself as an extremely toxic patient and went for a good and laxative combination salad as discussed in the *Mucusless Diet*. For a GI track with less toxicity, fruit is preferable. Again, in the early days, I learned to break it with a salad and would then get into some serious transitional meals including raw and cooked vegetables. I would then move toward a default diet of fruit juice for breakfast, fruit meal at lunch, and a transitional meal at night. I found this to be an important stage of my transition, as I was able to systematically begin permanently eliminating my addiction to mucus-forming foods. Once you feel that you are over major humps, like you could never eat or crave meat and dairy again, then fruit is advisable.

Transitioning Back into Eating

Brother Air broke his first 9½-month fast with a piece of watermelon, which put him to sleep immediately. After watching how he functioned after this, I decided that I would do a slow transition from juice to solid fruit over a long period of time when I did my first long fast. During the transition, there was a time when the line between juice and solid food was blurred, as my juices got thicker and became more like smoothies. By the time I ate my first salad, my intestines were ready.

Another more advanced option is to shift from fruit juice to juice and solid fruits. This is more of a mucusless fruitarian program or fruit fast. In the early days, I could fast on fruit juice, but solid fruit would make me crave mucus, which is why I advocate jumping into a progressive transitional program. This is one of the fundamental issues that I see with many "raw-food" advocates. They try to skip over the cooked, mucusless vegetable phases and often end up strung out on fatty nuts and avocados. Or worse, go back to meat.

These are just some examples of possible approaches to breaking a fast. Your own condition and goals should help you decide. Is your goal to get deep into a transition period or to only briefly break the fast and return back to fasting? Do you aspire to spend some time totally mucusless after your fast? In either case, an enema is highly advisable to help pull the toxic waste out.

Well done with the fast. You did not know it, but Bro Air, Baby Babaji, you, and I were all fasting at the same time. Strong vibes!

Peace, Love, and Breath!

-Prof. Spira

Mucus-Lean Menus for Terrible Mucus Cravings

Sent by Samantha Claire on December 20, 2011

AHHHHHHHHHHHH! I just want to scream. Coming off the fast=complete fail. Well, not a complete fail. I made sure I lined my stomach with fruits and veggies before I lined it with garbage. Yuk! Peanut butter and jelly sandwiches, I had a cookie my mom made, oatmeal. Not terrible stuff, but I definitely was not armed and have nasal congestion (which wasn't even part of the elimination because I wasn't congested with anything!).

At this time of my day, I am just going to finish what I have started but end it with a bean salad I got from the Greek international food store.

I shall keep trucking. I just wasn't prepared, even though you wrote me this wonderful piece. I still felt lost and confused and grabbed what I could when my appetite came back.

Are you still fasting?

-Sam

Spira's Response:

Sent by Prof. Spira on December 22, 2011

Sounds like you're ready to hear more about the nitty gritty of the transition. I usually do not talk much about mucus-lean transitional menus until someone has cleansed for a while. In this stage, I had to confront old cravings from my past and ancient cravings from my ancestors. One minute I'm thinking about pizza, and the next, African buffalo and gruel, which I've not eaten in this lifetime. My salvation was to find mucus-lean menus that satisfied the craving with as little damage as possible. I would often go to the store and walk around looking at different foods and imagine the effect they would have on me. How will it eliminate? What kind of mucus will this create in my intestines? How high (stimulated) will it make me? Do I crave it and why?

I will give you a few of the combinations that helped me along with approaches I've observed others use. I do not strongly recommend or suggest avoiding these. Just tuck the ideas away for what I refer to as the "crack head" days when you are in the supermarket craving insane stuff.

If you don't crave or need any of these, and can go straight into a raw mucusless program, then go for it. However, I've yet to see anyone not pass through some version of this transitional period and sustain a long-term, mucus-free lifestyle.

To get through this period, I had to adopt a survivalist, "by any means necessary" attitude. Nothing was going to prevent me from practicing the diet at its highest possible level. I drew my strongest inspiration from John Coltrane and endeavored to practice the diet on the level he practiced music. I mention this only to convey the challenge of this path.

Okay, now for the nasty:

You are familiar with the cleaner menus: combination salads, fruit, raw and steamed starchless veggies, etc., which are the mainstays.

Spira's Early Transitional Menus

When I first got into the diet, I ate a nice amount of raisin bran with soy milk. When I was getting off meat, I could crush a bunch of cereal with some wheat toast and soy butter. I would try to add extra raisins whenever possible. I did experiment with some of the different flavors of organic cereals, but did not want to get too strung out on them. The enemas and transition eventually made it too uncomfortable for me to eat this combination. Early on, I developed habits of good food combination and did not mix juicy fruit anywhere near mucus.

Another early transition menu that helped me get off dairy was cottage cheese, dates, applesauce, and brown sugar. If I ever have a craving for pie or sweets, hit with this and get ready to be high as a kite. Again, I could not handle cottage cheese for too long because the enemas considerably cleaned my intestines.

The mucusless menu that followed this was **Baked Banana Surprise**, with baked bananas, applesauce, dates, and brown sugar. To bake the bananas, I wrapped bananas in tinfoil (with skin on) and baked at about 415 for 15-20 min. You should see warm banana juice start to drip from the sides. Take the banana meat and combine with other ingredients. I've eaten pie and cakes from the best bakers in the world, and this crushes them all. Make this for your family and see their toes curl up.

104

One terrible craving that I had to deal with was potato chips. In the beginning, I got chips from the natural food section of the supermarket. This was one addiction that did not go away just because it made me sick. Every time I ate it, I would crush the whole bag and then feel horrid. Yet, I would be back the next day. I tried sweet potato chips, but did not like the brand that they sold. The work that I was doing in other areas of my diet eventually helped me get off of white potato chips. However, I did get into Sun Chips pretty bad. Corn chips also became a terrible addiction that lasted a long time.

Transitioning off Fast Food

Different kinds of cooked beans became a personal mucus-lean staple. The last days of my fast-food career consisted of 89¢ bean burritos with no cheese from "Taco Hell." I would crush several burritos and a bag of Sun Chips like it was going out of style, which fortunately it was. I eventually moved to buying cans of "Taco Bell vegetarian" refried beans and made concoctions at home. Onion, garlic, and olive oil sautés mixed with warm refried beans started to taste far better than anything I'd ever eaten at a "Mexican" restaurant. Warm some corn chip discs (whatever they are called), and it was over. Would even toast the discs, add beans with onions and garlic on top, broil for a few minutes, and go crazy. Although highly addicting, I noticed that the bean meals seemed to eliminate well without leaving behind too much mucus waste.

Bean Feasts

Another bean excursion was my gourmet bean soup/stew. I would fix the sauté, then combine with freshly juiced carrots, celery, and garlic (optional). Let the juice simmer and then put in a lot of beans. Kidney, black, northern, whatever I had. At first, I used the cheap store-bought brands saturated in corn syrup, but moved toward cleaner beans as I became more conscious. This meal was interesting because it filled me up, got me high, but did not hurt my stomach too badly. It was also less addictive, in that I did not turn into "crack head man" the next day. It also eliminated well.

Vegetarian chili also was big for a while. Fantastic brand chili mix would whoop me pretty good. I would also make my own with a bunch of cooked beans, tomatoes, tomato sauces, and spices. A big salad, chili, and about three slices of 100-percent-wheat toast with soy butter put me on the level.

Nature Burger

Speaking of Fantastic brand, I got crazy with their "Nature Burger." This was an item that Brother Air suggested and allowed his family to deal with. I got out a lot of my cravings with this stuff. I had a crazy craving for condiments with it, especially mayonnaise. I went to the natural food section and picked up non-egg versions (Nayonaise, I think). As a rule of thumb, I usually managed to stay away from all things with vinegar, except for these periods of intensive mucus craving. Ketchup and mustard also made brief appearances.

Messing with Soy Products

I also messed with some of the soy products in this mode. Go Lean soy burger meat was made into patties or put into tomato sauces. Soy lunchmeats were put on top of salads or even cooked with sauté. In fact, soy ham, turkey, and pepperoni sautéed and put onto toast with soy butter and mayo kicked my butt for a while (Cooked Dagwood lunchmeat sandwich with all meats, several kinds of cheese, and extra mayo from Penn Station used to be one of my favorite meals). Such soy items could also find their way on top of some vegetarian pizza.

Getting off Meat with 100-Percent-Wheat Spaghetti

By far, my staple mucus meal was 100-percent-wheat spaghetti with a ton of tomato sauce. My tomato sauces were almost like vegetable stews, and as my pallet got cleaner, I did not want the spaghetti anymore. Steamed broccoli and cabbage with tomato sauce became the rule, and this meal helped eliminate cravings of some of the stuff above. It was a wonderful transitional meal because any kind of baked starchless vegetable could fit in the mix. Baked zucchini, acorn squash, etc. were nice additions. Baked sweet potatoes with soy butter and wheat toast rounded out this meal.

Brother Air got me hip to his natural peanut butter and jelly on wheat toast. He had a long addiction to it, but it helped move him forward. I got into it for a while, but could not handle the combination for too long. Also, in general, I advise against mixing fruit (jelly), fats, and starches. But, the meal is there if you need it.

Periods of Refined Fruit Eating

At this point, I learned that no matter how badly I ate, I would need to adhere to good combinations. As bad as the menus above became, my fruit eating on the other side was often and usually mono in nature; free from combination and experimentation. If I had apples for lunch, that was it. Pineapple, that's it. Oranges, that's it. And I would not overeat or stuff myself with fruit. I wanted my fruit eating to be as refined as possible because I knew that I would spend more time in the future as a fruit eater. I wanted to leave my bad habits behind in the cooked, mucus-lean world and allow my mucus-free world to be as unsullied as possible. As a result, I opted to stay away from raw-food cookbooks and many such concoctions. When I'm eating raw, I like to be mucusless and mono-fruit (this is why many raw foodists find me to be no fun). I avoided getting into raw chocolates, candies, and other foods in that direction. I mention this because it sheds light on the impact of my long-term intentions. I knew that the above menus would not last forever and wanted to move forward ASAP. As I transformed my body, each addiction was systematically cleared away. Yet, my long-term aspirations were that of a mono-raw-fruitarian.

After doing a lot of short-term fasting in these periods, I realized that if I could grab ahold of a long fast, I could ascend into a different dimension. Like a warp zone in a video game, I theorized that I could float over years of pain to higher levels. There are no shortcuts, yet I recognized that fasting is the omnipotent healing force of the Universe and that its power is accessible. After seeing Brother Air fast for almost a year, I knew that it was possible. I never *tried* to fast, but I knew that my body would present me with the opportunity. The question was, would I be mentally prepared? After a while, I noticed that my body was advancing faster than my mind could follow. As I felt addictions slipping from my body, my mind started to panic. "This stuff is real and actually works." On a certain level, the mind/ego needs the chaos of mucus-addiction to remain relevant and in power. At this point, I endeavored to not give into my mind's will. Yet, if I craved something, I would eat it with no guilt, knowing that eventually I would not be able to physically tolerate it.

In general, I would fast in the morning, eat a large fruit meal or fruit juice meal in the afternoon, and a vegetable/mucus-lean meal in the evening. When large amounts of mucus were being eliminated, I got in the good habit of fasting. If I can remember, I think my first juice fast

107

was on a generic brand's 100 percent grape juice. This stuff was a revelation to me from where I was coming from. Later, as I became cleaner, I could only tolerate Welch's 100 percent grape juice. For the past 6 months, I've had no store bought juice and have only juiced with my juicer.

Overall, I'm an advocate for a long, progressive, rational transition toward the highest dietetic levels attainable, limited only by one's own constitution.

Being Real about the Transition

This is the first time that I've shared my transition with someone with this much detail. As mentioned above, I do not advocate or recommend any of these menus. I offer them only to put things into perspective. Most people do not like to share these kinds of details in books or lectures. Dietetic writing and talking-head gurus usually focus on the way things would play out in a perfect world. And many tend to leave out the grittier elements of their journey. Such altruistic ideals are useful to expand the psyche of an aspirant, yet they can lead to guilt if not attained. Raw fruitarianism with fasting is an altruistic and attainable goal. But the individual path that one takes to achieve it on a long-term basis is not perfect. The biographies of pioneers like Arnold Ehret and even Robert Morse show what happens if a long transition is not adhered to. It has been said that Robert Morse broke his 5-year fruit diet with a piece of fish. From what I gather, he did 6 months eating nothing but vine-ripened oranges and then lived as a hermit in national parks for about 5 years eating nothing but fruit. Why did he crave fish? After 5 years of a fruit or mucusless diet, meat cravings should be gone. In Morse's case, it seems that he did not transition very long before jumping into an all fruit diet. If Morse had spent 15 years transitioning, would he have been able to sustain a fruit level permanently? This is by no means a criticism, but an observation. Ehret also did an extended fruit fast of 2 years. The story is that he traveled around Europe and the Middle East during the intensive fruit-fasting period. When he broke the fast, he conducted his blood-clotting experiment, which ended with him eating meat.

My question is, how long would they have needed to transition to be permanently mucusless or fruitarian? Again, I point out these stories not to criticize but to consider them as vital information given to us by great pioneers that can help us avoid such potholes in our journeys.

Still Fasting

I am still fasting. I am in raw-fruit and fruit-juice fasting mode. Freshly juiced grapes and blackberries have been the staple, with a little lemon juice. Recently, apples have been added to the juice to make it last longer as money gets scarce. I also had some days of only apple juice, which were interesting. When juicing and eating fruit, I have a few mission figs followed by a handful of blackberries or grapes. I have not craved a salad or green drink in a long while; but if I do, I will break the fruit fast. My plan would be to eat a couple salads and then get back to fruit, which is easier said than done. But it's been all fruit for several months. This is my first long-term, sub-acid fruit (grapes, berries) fast. My former fasting usually consisted mostly of citrus fruit juices, oranges, and pineapple.

I hope that this helps. When I was getting into the diet, I hung with Bro Air and his family all the time learning about what everyone ate. As I learned more about the details of everyone's transition, I felt more confident and equipped to transition myself safely and successfully.

Stay strong and keep on transitioning!

Peace, Love, and Breath!

-Spira

Vintage video of me at Brother Air's house talking about my transition. I had been into the diet about 1 year at the time of the video: "Dialog with Brother Air: Spira and Tacorah talk about Arnold Ehret's Mucusless Diet Healing System" (visit http://bit.ly/tacorah). *Taken from a day-long round table discussion about the Mucusless Diet Healing System with Brother Air in November 2003.*

Family Issues

Sent by Samantha Claire on February 10, 2011

My family just doesn't get it.

I'm so close to bursting.

My dad was supposed to take me to a wholesaler (which is in a neighborhood known for its heavy prostitution activity). I can only go place an order and pick up between 5 a.m. and 9 a.m. (a decent prostitution hour), and my dad canceled today. He then said next Friday we'll go. NEXT FRIDAY! I am broke and in tremendous need of oranges to fast. I feel DISGUSTING and need to FAST. I wanted to make freshly squeezed OJ for the next week. But, that has to wait because they don't understand the importance of an abundance of fruit.

Nor do they want to.

So I am off to get my driver permit. Step 1. I cannot depend on anyone anymore. But I need to cleanse, but cannot. So damn frustrating.

Yesterday I broke down and cried, and I thought today would be better, but I woke up ANGRY. Damn, I don't wake up angry either, that's just not in my character. But I don't know.

The damn health food store wants $100 for a box of oranges, whereas as the wholesale place wants $28.

GRRRRRRrrrrrrrrr.

Spira's Response:

Sent by Prof. Spira on February 10, 2011

That's a rough situation. I'm glad to hear that you'll be getting your driver license. That independence is crucial! It's weird, because there seems to be a fine line between accepting much-needed help from family and closing yourself off from them for protection during these intense periods of healing. GRRRRRRrrrrrrrr indeed! Keep your head up and keep on pushin'! If stuff gets super deep, don't hesitate to let me know if you need anything.

Peace, Love, and Breath!

-Spira

Sent by Samantha Claire on February 10, 2011

I know. It's just so frustrating because I always get to this threshold and cannot push past it. This happened to me last May, this past December, and now. I was going to supply myself up with massive amounts of oranges to cleanse. What do you do in this situation? Not fast when you know you should? Not eat juicy fruits even though it doesn't feel good otherwise?

Sent by Prof. Spira on February 11, 2011

Survivalist Mode

That's a good question. In real hard situations, I get deep into a survivalist mode and find a way to get what I need by any means necessary. Each situation might be different, but the mental processes are the same. In your case, is it possible to call some friends who have cars that might be willing to drive you to the wholesaler? Are there nearby stores where you can talk with the managers or owners to see if you can buy cases from them at a discount? I've done this kind of thing many times, especially with mom/pop stores, Mexican groceries, or street vendors—often for bulk lemons and oranges.

One rule I made for myself was there would be no compromise if I felt I needed to fast, etc. For me, everything in my life revolves around the diet. With that kind of submission, I've found that I often don't have all I "want," but I'm given what I "need." In the most extreme of situations, I might just water- or lemon-water fast until things around me get better. It is like the deeper I'm prepared to go, the more things around me shift to help out. And the help often came from the oddest of places.

With that said, all we can do is the best we can. If all you have access to right now is a limited supply of mucusless fruits and vegetables from a local market, then you could maybe hover there until you can get the fruit you need for your deeper cleanse. At this point, you can't go wrong in finding a mucusless groove.

Peace, Love, and Breath!

-Spira

Check out this video:

Plato's Allegory of the Cave—Claymation Cartoon (visit www.bit.ly/cave-allegory)

I love this allegory. Particularly the part where the newly liberated soul attempts to share the good news of freedom with his friends and family, only to be misunderstood, dismissed, viewed as insane, and even threatened with death. This aspect is particularly well-portrayed in the claymation version.

Plato's Cave—animated version (visit http://bit.ly/cave-allegory)

Yet, as suggested in the animated version, the liberated soul is still obligated to make an effort to help elevate his or her enslaved brothers and sisters, despite their fears, resentments, and attachments to their own bondage.

Etymological Explorations

Sent by Samantha Claire on May 12, 2011

I feel so good! I went to Chinatown and bought 5 pounds of grapes at $1 a pound. I know they are sprayed and jacked up with crap, but I need them. And at $1/lb, who can resist?

I do have a question. You are always researching and finding obscure information about the truths behind what we eat and what are in out foods and etc., etc., etc. I am wondering if you have a good source of where you research or HOW you research.

ALSO, could you send me some stuff (anything?) that exposes the truth (whatever that may be)?

I love you!

-Sam

Spira's Response:

Sent by Prof. Spira on March 22, 2011

We are on the same page. 99¢-a-pound grapes have been wonderful!

Nutrition

That is a great question. Below I will outline my initial process for researching concepts. First, I might begin with a concept or word that I want to understand better. Let's consider *nutrition*. I will initially begin with a hypothesis or thesis statement of what I intend to test. In light of Arnold Ehret's critique of nutrition, I offer the following thesis:

> **Hypothesis:** The foundation on which Western dietetic and medical science is based is wrong.

Then I consider a proposition, or what I think my research will ultimately reveal:

> **Proposition:** A critical examination of the historical origins of theories related to nutrition will reveal egregious flaws in the logic and science of the newly invented concepts.

Then I ask myself some questions:

What is the origin of the term; who coined it? What was the socio-cultural circumstance under which the concept was created? In the case of nutrition, we know that early medical researchers assumed that humans are omnivorous. In other words, they assumed that their dietetic practices were natural and endeavored to develop a science to support these claims.

Then I look up the etymology of the key terms related to the concept. I also may consider various definitions of the word.

Nutrition—1550s, from L. nutritionem (nom. nutritio) "a nourishing," from nutrire "nourish, [to] suckle" (see nourish) ["Nutrition," accessed from Etymolonline.com]

Above, we see that the original notion of nutrition had to do with nourishment, particularly that of a mother nursing her baby, i.e., to suckle. Thus, it can be seen that the original concept of nutrition did not have to do with a notion that the body needs a particular kind of chemistry to survive. But it was more of a natural concept connected to the means by which a person, especially an infant, sustains itself.

Sometimes a string of related words will be revealed. I then examine their etymologies:

Nourish—late 13c., "to bring up, nurture" (a child, a feeling, etc.), from O.Fr. norriss-, stem of norrir (Fr. nourir), from L. nutrire "to feed, nurse, foster, support, preserve," from *nutri (older form of nutrix "nurse"), lit. "she who gives suck," from PIE root *(s)nu- "flow, let flow," hence "to suckle" (cf. Skt. snauti "she drips, gives milk," Gk. nao "I flow") ["Nourish," accessed from Etymolonline.com].

A very interesting etymological find, indeed! As you can see, *nourish* is connected directly with "nurturing" or bringing up children. "Nutri" derives from "nurse," or literally "she who gives suck." Yet again, the origins of this concept are rooted in a concept of nature. Yet, to gain a deeper understanding, it is important to now investigate the other relevant words. When I search *nurture* on Etymolonline.com, a list of related words appear, including: nurture, nurturance, nourish, and nature. Consider nurture:

Nurture—early 14c. (n.), "breeding, upbringing," from O.Fr. nourriture "nourishment," from L.L. nutritia (see nursery). The verb meaning "to feed or nourish" is attested from early 15c.

Late 13c., "restorative powers of the body, bodily processes; powers of growth;" from O.Fr. nature, from L. natura "course of things, natural character, the universe," lit. "birth," from natus "born," pp. of nasci "to be born," from PIE *gene- "to give birth, beget" (see genus).

Nature—From late 14c. as "creation, the universe;" also "heredity, birth, hereditary circumstance; essential qualities, innate disposition" (e.g. human nature); "nature personified, Mother Nature." Nature and nurture have been contrasted since 1874.

Nature should be avoided in such vague expressions as "a lover of nature,""poems about nature." Unless more specific statements follow, the reader cannot tell whether the poems have to do with natural scenery, rural life, the sunset, the untouched wilderness, or the habits of squirrels." (Strunk & White, "The Elements of Style," 3rd ed., 1979, cited in "Nature," accessed from Etymolonline.com)

Once I have a better understanding of the origins and lineage of the words associated with the concept in question, I look to encyclopedias for a basic history. Wikipedia is a good source to do preliminary research. Although you would normally not want to cite material from Wikipedia in a formal essay, most articles have a comprehensive list of sources that you could follow up with. But, for a quick analysis, Wikipedia works well. Keep in mind that I read all such histories very critically. As I read, I constantly challenge the validity of what I am reading. I consider the belief system (paradigm) of the people who wrote what I'm reading, and the socio-cultural context in which they exist.

Consider the following excerpt from the "History of Nutrition":

Around 475 BC, Anaxagoras stated that food is absorbed by the human body and therefore contained "homeomerics" (generative components), suggesting the existence of nutrients. Around 400 BC, Hippocrates said, "Let food be your medicine and medicine be your food."

In the sixteenth century, scientist and artist Leonardo da Vinci compared metabolism to a burning candle. In 1747, Dr. James Lind, a physician in the British Navy, performed the first scientific nutrition experiment, discovering that lime juice saved sailors who had been at sea for years from scurvy, a deadly and painful bleeding disorder. The discovery was ignored for 40 years, after which British sailors became known as "limeys." The essential Vitamin C within lime juice would not be identified by scientists until the 1930s. ["Nutrition" accessed from Wikipedia]

Although I will not give a full analysis here, I immediately notice that the "lime juice" cure for scurvy may have been misattributed to solving a "vitamin" deficiently instead of a condition of severe mucus constipation (i.e., stagnant lymphatic system). We understand that lemon and lime juice are the strongest detoxifiers. Considering the fact that many of the sick sailors probably lost their appetite, it is possible that lime-juice fasting is what truly helped them heal. In other words, healing occurs when waste is loosened and removed, not by adding some kind of mineral.

Around 1770, Antoine Lavoisier, the "Father of Nutrition and Chemistry," discovered the details of metabolism, demonstrating that the oxidation of food is the source of body heat. In 1790, George Fordyce recognized calcium as necessary for fowl survival. In the early nineteenth century, the elements carbon, nitrogen, hydrogen, and oxygen were recognized as the primary components of food, and methods to measure their proportions were developed.

In 1816, François Magendie discovered that dogs fed only carbohydrates and fat lost their body protein and died in a few weeks, but dogs also fed protein survived, identifying protein as an essential dietary component. In 1840, Justus Liebig discovered the chemical makeup of carbohydrates (sugars), fats (fatty acids), and proteins (amino acids.) In the 1860s, Claude Bernard discovered that body fat can be synthesized from carbohydrate and protein, showing that the energy in blood glucose can be stored as fat or as glycogen. ["Nutrition," accessed from Wikipedia]

Above, each one of the so-called "discoveries" could be deeply researched, analyzed, and critiqued using Ehret's frame of reference. But, for all of them, it must be understood that they built their theories on top of other theories that were erroneous. Again, consider Magendie's sadistic experiment on starving dogs. Dogs that were fed protein survived, whereas dogs that only drank water died. He reasoned that the dogs that died first did so because they lacked a certain nitrogenous substance. Yet, we understand the dogs that were fed only water died because their elimination was much too aggressive. They did not die because they lacked a nitrogenous substance (i.e., protein), but because they loosened too much waste into their bloodstreams too rapidly. This resulted in oxygen not being able to get into the bloodstream, and the dog essentially drowned in its own waste. The dogs that were fed experienced a slowing down of their body's elimination.

Protein Theory

The etymology of protein also reveals its fallacy:

Protein—1844, from Fr. protéine, coined 1838 by Dutch chemist Gerhard Johan Mulder (1802-1880), perhaps on suggestion of Berzelius, from Gk. proteios "the first quality [principle]," from protos "first" (see proto-). Originally a theoretical substance thought to be essential to life; the modern use as a general name for a class of bodies is from German, used thus in English from 1907. ["Protein," accessed from Etymolonline.com]

For a more detailed analysis, the above may be cross-referenced with a standard article on the "History of Protein." But, how absurd is this theory: The premise that "protein" is the "first or primary principle" to life? If there is a first principle to life, would it not be air? So, we have an extremely problematic term and theory that is based upon a wrong interpretation of why tortured and murdered dogs perished. Such is the medieval thinking that persists to this day.

***

Much more analysis could and should go into these topics. The foundation on which Western medical and dietetic science was developed should be ripped apart and reconsidered based upon the premise that humans are air-eating frugivores. As more people begin to understand and experience Vitality = Power - Obstruction, such theories will become futile. Nutritional concepts like protein will be exposed for what they really are—sophisticated excuses to eat pus and mucus.

Peace, Love, and Breath!

-Prof. Spira

Calorie Myth

Sent by Prof. Spira on March 24, 2011

Okay, time to take the gloves off. I'm disheartened to hear folks be so befuddled by this calorie myth nonsense. It might be time to go through each one of these commonly held theories and deconstruct them. Using the methods I showed you above, it took me about 20 minutes to put this together. I kept it short because I might get feedback from dietitians/doctors who want to defend the theory, which will push me to further refine my analysis. Yet, this is basically my writing/research process. I might post this on a forum to get feedback, but would not publish it to a wide audience yet. I'm always interested to see what happens when I start to turn up the heat in such forums! Get it . . . heat/calorie/joule (nerd joke).

> (@ 10:40 from www. bit.ly/dr-morse-calorie) **Calorie myth deconditioning lesson**: "I don't deal with calories, I just don't even put my head there, and I don't think that any other animal does [either] . . ." Thank you Dr. Morse!

The calorie (c. 1865 deriving from the Latin calor, gen. caloris, i.e. "heat") is one of the most erroneous theories to emerge from Western dietetic theory. What is known as "food energy" is defined as the amount of energy obtained from food available through cellular respiration. It should be understood that the founders of this theory based such concepts on their own eating habits. The assumption was that meat, dairy, and starches were obviously the staples of omnivorous Homo sapiens. Such a theory would help to support and rationalize eating in this manner. Yet, as many of us know today through our own experiences, humans are far from biologically being omnivorous. Humans, as a tropical frugivorous species, survived for years without trying to measure the amount of heat it takes to raise the temperature of one kilogram of water by one degree Celsius (one "large" calorie). Such thinking has nurtured a fundamentally flawed notion of nutrition and metabolism. What Western dietitians view as "energy" from food, is nothing more than "stimulation." Energy, i.e. true vitality in the human body, exists only in an internal environment that is free of acidic wastes, mucus, and uneliminated, toxic, foreign matters. And how is it possible for a so-called calorimeter to incinerate food like a human body? It simply does not. The concept of calories is, at best, not useful; and the fanaticism surrounding it unfortunate.

*Worry not what a calorimeter reads,
but consider the amount of mucus waste
a particular food breeds.*

Peace, Love, and Breath!

-Prof. Spira

VOLUME TWO (Intermediate Literature)

Chapter 4—Practical Analysis and Philosophical Inquiry Inspired

by the Mucusless Diet

Art of the Transition Part 1: A Response to Stanley Bass and Others on the Art of Ehret's Transition Diet

When one does a Google search on Arnold Ehret, an article named "Fruit: Friend or Foe" by Stanley Bass usually appears toward the top of the results. In the article, Bass reflects on his experimentation with fruit dieting and fasting. After being influenced by local naturopathic doctors at a young age and reading many authors from the Back-to-Nature/Natural-Hygienic movement, such as John Henry Tilden, Bass began to fervently experiment with radical dietary changes. He did intensive fruit-juice- and water-fasts without the necessary aid of a slow, rational transition. Later in his life, he, then a nutritionist, learned of Arnold Ehret's *Mucusless Diet Healing System*. However, his interpretation of Ehret's dynamic system was that humans are fundamentally frugivores. As many of his raw-fruitarian-aspiring peers before and after him had, he disregarded the proposition of the TRANSITION DIET, and tried to implement radical periods of all-fruit eating. He then experienced many negative symptoms, including bleeding of the gums and ultimately the loss of teeth. Later, adopting more of a raw-foodist approach, he lived on fruits, vegetables, nuts and avocados—the latter two being mucus-forming. It should be noted that at no point did Bass's description of his radical dietetic endeavors resemble a rational and effective application of Arnold Ehret's *Mucusless Diet Healing System*

121

Many students of the Back-to-Nature/Natural-Hygiene movement notice that many of the pioneering fruitarian thinkers went through intensive periods of elimination, which sometimes scared them away from their pursuit of natural living. Even worse, many of them reverted to the nutrition mythology of Western dietetic theory and blamed the fruit, or the lack of other nutrients, for their debilitating conditions. And today, many of those who claim to be "fruitarians," raw foodists, or vegans dive in to such diets head first and feel great for a while only to experience tremendous FALLS (i.e. intensive and potentially dangerous periods of elimination/detoxification). However, in every case that I've examined, an improper transition and/or misinterpretation of Ehret's work seems to be at the root of the problem. In most cases, people do not understand the fundamental importance and sophistication of THE TRANSITION DIET. The Art of the Transition is, indeed, one of the greatest of all arts that can be undertaken by human beings. Yet, as important as the transition is—like breath—it is greatly underdiscussed and misunderstood.

Although Ehret was a fruitarian thinker who asserted that a mono-fruit diet is the best for humans, he by no means suggested that people in our pathological condition can achieve such a level immediately without a considerable amount of dietary transition and PRACTICE of the *Mucusless Diet*. Many health seekers hear of fruitarianism and aspire to just jump right in without an extended period of transition. Using the *Mucusless Diet Healing System* as a means to save a terminally ill patient is different from using it as a transitional lifestyle to achieve superior health. The principles are the same, but they must be applied a bit differently by relatively able-bodied health seekers versus those who are chronically ill and on their deathbeds. Ehret wrote his articles, which resulted in the *Mucusless Diet Healing System* and *Rational Fasting*, geared toward saving the lives of deathly ill patients after his experiences saving thousands at his sanitariums. Meanwhile, he was experimenting with living the principles of his transition on a long-term basis. Such experiences greatly influenced his application of the healing system to his patients, who were basically only using it on a short-term basis to save their lives. The distinction between short- and long-term applications must be understood when learning to adapt the principles of the transition to achieving long-term goals.

How Long Will the Transition Take?

One question I often ask people to ponder is how long ago they think they had two fruitarian parents in their bloodline? We all have fruitarians in our bloodline, yet many of us must travel through some scary ancestral pus and mucus to get to them. This is where an intensive investigation into the history of your own bloodline and GI tract can help you to better understand how long it might take you to accomplish certain levels of physiological freedom. We all have various amounts of mucus constipation on the cellular level, and our transitions will look very different based upon our unique situations. My father is from Trinidad, where living on mangos from the trees outside—while not being able to afford much meat or anything else—was a reality of his childhood. In the islands, there was no one around trying to say that you need protein or that you cannot live off fruit. Mangos were on the trees and that is what was eaten by folks who did not have access to anything else; a totally different reality—one much closer to nature. Consequently, many elders on these islands do not resemble those I'm accustomed to seeing in the US, as they are often fundamentally healthier and seem to live much longer with fewer afflictions (which is quickly changing as KFC and Taco Hell become modern mainstays in such countries). At any rate, my father's childhood fruit eating certainly contributed in a positive way to my physiological aspirations of pursuing the *Mucusless Diet*. On the other hand, I was a particularly egregious omnivoric overeater of the worst kinds of mucus-forming foods, growing up 100 percent S.A.D. (Standard American Diet)! The latter situation forced me to become very studious and analytical about every facet of my transition. If I wanted to save myself, I knew that I would need to put serious thought into practicing the diet.

Intuition and Intellect

I feel right at home during periods of extended fruit eating, but in times of mucus-lean eating I have found that I have certain cravings that are particularly challenging to overcome. In those instances, my intuition is obstructed and I need to rely more on my own intellectual analysis. But, through detailed considerations of my own transitional process, based upon Ehret's principles, I have been able to make it through situations that may have otherwise derailed me. Given the attributes and challenges of my own bloodline, I learned that I need to allow for a good balance of intuition and intellect to be successful with practicing the mucusless diet. People who might start out physiologically cleaner

123

than I may have a far more advanced sense of intuition than I did when I began. Such individuals may not need to rely as heavily on their intellectual understanding of the process, but let their bodies guide the process the majority of the time. But for some of us who are not physiological geniuses, and who have gotten so far away from nature that they may not be able to "feel" the idea of the diet at all, intellect can save the day. Such individuals can cultivate and rely on their ability to think and reason.

When Brother Air first told me that he went a year eating nothing but fruit, I felt what he was saying deep in my soul. It touched me on a fundamental level. The proposition of fruit-eating humans uncovered a memory of who I really am and where I come from, which I had simply forgotten. As I continue to experience the transition first hand, this internal knowingness grows stronger and stronger. Brother Air says that he had a similar "ah-ha" experience when he read Lesson V of the *Mucusless Diet*. "Your body is an air-gas engine" touched him deeply. The mere suggestion uncovered an internal knowingness that sparked his intuition.

But for those who might not be able to "feel" Brother Air's news about fruit eating, fasting, air-gas engines, or mucusless diet, one's own internal Socratic dialogues of reason and rationality can help to better understand what can no longer be naturally "felt." Are humans frugivores? If it is possible for some primates to live on fruits, and humans are presumed to be the most "evolved," then why can humans not also live on fruit alone? If humans could eat only fruit, would it not be the most rational of diets—both physically and ethically? What process must mucus-eating humans go through to return to a fruit-based reality? Is it possible that mucus-forming foods are not only unnecessary for human life, but the very foundation of human illness? Given the fundamental errors in the history of scientific thought (paradigms—see Thomas Kuhn), to what extent is our modern understanding of metabolism and nutrition fundamentally flawed and dangerous? How did social, cultural, and political contexts influence the foundation of Western dietetic and medical theories? If breath is fundamental to life, and my nose periodically becomes constipated by mucus, can this process be viewed as an emergency signal from my body to stop eating mucus and FAST?

In addition to uncovering how reasonable and rational the propositions of the *Mucusless Diet* are, intellectual interrogation of the transitional process can greatly inform and enhance the decisions made by a practitioner. In the way that an aspiring composer may systematically analyze the music of other great composers, or a young painter work on a particular set of traditional and modern drawing techniques to enhance their skills, the *Mucusless Diet Healing System* practitioner can benefit from a vigorous analysis of the principles and processes of the transition diet. Overall, not unlike an improvising jazz musician, intuition and intellectual prowess can be joined by the aspiring health seeker to create a wonderful symphony of physiological art.

Unrealistic Perspectives

All in all, most people have an unrealistic perspective of how sick they are and how long it will take to permanently transition to higher levels of physiological liberation. After 2 years of living on fruit with intensive sessions of fasting, Ehret ended up eating meat again (resulting in his famous bloodletting experiment). This experience suggests that Ehret had much more transitioning to do to get to the point where eating meat would have not been an option. For me, eating meat is now like drinking Clorox bleach—it is just not a part of my world as food to potentially be eaten. After 5 years of living on mostly raw fruits, Dr. Robert Morse—a great modern-day healer, naturopath, and student/advocate of Ehret's work—broke his extended period of raw fasting with a piece of fish. His own reflections about the early days of his dietary change toward a raw, fruit-based reality indicate that he did not spend a long time slowly transitioning. I mean not to criticize these pioneers, but reference their experiences so that we might learn from them and put into proper perspective how long and challenging a rational transition really is.

Stanley Bass was way too filthy to try to do the kind of extended fruit fasting that he did without expecting some intensive, and even dangerous, results. No one told him not to eat mucus-free vegetables in a systematic manner with fruit. No one told him that it is a sin to use cooked, mucus-free vegetable menus to control and SLOW DOWN his elimination (at least not Ehert). No one said that even some cooked, mucus-lean menus are prohibited during the beginning of such a lofty dietetic undertaking.

Learning to control one's elimination is fundamental to the Art of the Transition. Bass, Fry, and many other fruitarian thinkers and aspirants tried to progress faster than their mind and bodies would allow. Ehret often said, "Nature's mills grind slowly," and he clearly says that he does not recommend extended fruit or water fasting for most patients—especially for those who have never been through any kind of transition diet. Yet, many assume that Ehret means radical fruit and water fasting, which he does not. Ehret's healing system is not immediate raw foodism, mono-fruit diet, or irrational, extended water fasting, but a SYSTEM that coordinates the use of raw and cooked mucusless and mucus-lean menus—in concert with short- and long-term periods of RATIONAL FASTING—to safely and effectively transition off of all mucus-forming foods. Yes, a raw-fruit-mono-diet is identified to be supreme; yet we must earn this level of excellence, not overnight, but only after having paid reparations for the wrong that we and our relatives have done to our bodies all the days of our lives. The key to sustaining the diet on a long-term basis is mastery of the Art of Transition. Whether it is through intuition, intellect, spiritual awakening, or scientific understanding, emancipating oneself from eating pus and mucus must be a top priority for those interested in physiological freedom. And after generations of mucus-eating ancestors, it will simply not happen overnight. There is no shortcut around the transition. As Brother Air often says, "You can be on the transition diet for more than 30 years if you need to be, but you will still be here."

Peace, Love, and Breath!

Prof. Spira

This article began as a discussion on the Prof. Arnold Ehret Facebook Support Group. I would like to thank all members of the group for fostering such a high level of discourse about the *Mucusless Diet*.

How Long Was Arnold Ehret on Raw Foods?

-Baby and Earl (Ehret Support Group Member and rawinspirationdaily.com webmaster)

It cannot be said with certainty how long Ehret remained mucusless and raw. Ehret is best known for his series of extended fasts, which were scientifically monitored by Swiss government officials, where a fast of 49 days remained the world record for several decades. Suffice it to say, many people were completely blown away by Ehret's monitored fasts. Yet, as with those of us who push ourselves physiologically to uncover deeper levels of unrealized human potential, many health seekers thought that they should be able to accomplish similar feats without years of transition or study. But Ehret's demonstration was not meant to be a public spectacle—like a David Blaine trick—but to challenge and show that the fundamental reasoning upon which the burgeoning Western medical establishment was being based is fundamentally erroneous. His influence among medical professionals in Europe during the late 1800s was tremendous, as his work split early researchers into Ehretists and non-Ehretists. In addition to these officially monitored fasts, we have accounts of Ehret's own experiences weaved into his articles/books about mucusless diet and fasting. One of the most notable accounts is of his 2 years of intensive fasting and fruit diet. During this period, he traveled (I believe mostly by foot or bicycle) with a friend around Europe and Northern Africa. These accounts show off his physical prowess as he talks about advanced feats of strength and vitality.

There are also observations written by close colleagues and others. Ehret became a role model for early Back to Naturists, as he was known for living in the woods for long periods on fruit, doing 8-hour-long daily sun baths, and exercising. But how long he maintained these high levels is not known. Kind of like Dr. Robert Morse's 5 years living and fasting in the wilderness, or Brother Air's multiple 9½-month-long juice fasts, retrospective accounts about the experience survive, but detailed ethnographic or scientific renderings of exactly what went on are not well recorded. From what I've gathered from the writings I've read, I think that Ehret was in the process of truly adapting the mucusless diet as a sustainable lifestyle, and not only as the short-term cure that it was to many of the thousands of patients he saved in his sanitarium.

As to the specific point of being raw, Ehret's writings focus primarily on transitioning toward, and sustaining, a mucusless (mucus-free) diet, while being "raw" is assumed for the higher-level periods of fruit eating and fasting. For Ehret, being raw was not enough, as some popular raw items can be mucus-forming. Yet, little mention is made about the amount, if any, of cooked mucusless or mucus-lean menus he ate when he was not fasting or eating just fruits. In fact, the only place that I recall him really talking about eating what I assume to be cooked food was during his famous bloodletting experiment. Further, many of the mucus-lean menus from the *Mucusless Diet* were presumably added by Fred Hirsch, as Ehret's readers wanted to see examples of mucus-lean transitional menus. They were items used to help heal some of the sickest patients in the world, but it is not clear the degree to which Ehret ate of such menus.

In time, as more of his untranslated and unpublished works become available, additional details about specific periods when Ehret was mucusless and raw may be uncovered. As one can imagine, there are many questionable writings and negative rumors about Ehret and his lifestyle. My attitude toward most of them is that I do not, and will never, know with 100 percent certainty about Ehret's daily practices because I was not there. In my opinion, such personal accounts are only useful to the degree that they help others experience the truth for themselves. I have not read it in a long time, but when initially confronted with "The Story of My Life," supposedly dictated by Ehret to a close female companion, it just did not sound like Ehret to me. It came across more as a piece of fan fiction than a true account. To this day, its validity is quite unclear.

In sum, undeniable proof exists of Ehret's extended fasting experiments and miraculous healings at his sanitarium. But it is unclear what his longest stint of being mucusless or raw was before his untimely and suspicious death.

Peace, Love, and Breath!

Prof. Spira

Also see: www.mucusfreelife.com/world-record-for-going-without-food/

Arnold Ehret and Raw Foodism

August 11, 2011

Greetings Brothers and Sisters!

I wanted to take a moment and explore the notion of "raw food" through Ehret's lens. In this age of "-isms" (raw foodism, veganism, vegetarianism, fruitarianism, etc.), the work of Ehret continues to challenge both medical and naturopathic philosophies. The foundation of Western medical and dietetic theory rests upon the notion of "nutrition," that is, the idea that one must assimilate elements from food to survive. One of the most revolutionary aspects of Ehret's work is his dismissal of the "nutrition" theory and observation of Vitality=Power-Obstruction as the principle for life. Why do we eat? According to Ehret, we do not eat to gain energy, build strength, etc., but to eliminate waste. As waste is eliminated, real vitality is possible. This is not the "stimulation" that occurs when mucus-formers are consumed. Why do we breathe? Our bodies are air-gas engines that subsist off of air.

Consider this excerpt from the *Mucusless Diet Healing System*:

At present among the vegetarian health-seekers, "raw-food diet" is in fashion. No doubt it represents great progress, but the arguments are partly wrong and lead to mistaken and fanatic extremes.

They claim all cooking destroys food values, but it should be said properly: "Wrong cooking destroys HEALING value qualities (efficiency) of foods and can even cause them to become acid forming." The "raw food" experts hint on the same wrong stress as all others, i.e., the higher food value.

The entire effect or benefit from raw food is the rough fiber of uncooked vegetables which relieves constipation and acts as an ideal "mucus broom" in the intestines. I do not believe that the human body assimilates "food-value vegetables" such as cauliflower, asparagus, turnips, potatoes, or from uncooked cereals. After a certain beneficial mechanical cleansing of the bowels through these raw foods, the one-sided raw-food eater lacks, in fact, the most important food substance, and that is grape or fruit sugar, unless they eat sufficient fruits.

Significant and instructive is this experiment: Put a lemon in a moderate dry heat a few minutes, and it becomes sweet—like an orange. You develop grape sugar, but let it bake a little too long, or if cooked, it becomes bitter. On the same principle, all vegetables when baked improve by developing the more or less starch they contain into grape-sugar. This is true of carrots, beets, turnips, cauliflower, etc.

Raw fruits, and if desired, raw green-leafy vegetables, form the ideal food for humans. That is the mucusless diet. But the mucusless diet as a healing system uses raw, rough vegetables for their cleansing qualities; baked ones as food; and baked and stewed fruits AS A LESS AGGRESSIVE DISSOLVER of poisons and mucus to MODERATE THE ELIMINATION IN SEVERE CASES. That is one of the most important principles of the system, a point the raw-food fanatic ignores entirely. Eating raw potatoes, raw cereals, and unfired pies, is, in my opinion, absurd and worse than if they are carefully baked, which means developing the starch into at least partly digestible gluten and grape sugar. ("Confusions in Dietetics, Part 2" in MDHS)

CONFUSION IN DIETETICS (Part 3) LESSON XIII

After this severe critique of all important dietetics, I must admit that I do not deny that all of them have, and have done, considerable good towards the development of the dietetical solution of the food problem and healing of diseases by diet.

Reviewing the entire development during the past 25 years, this fact remains: With the progress of chemistry, medical experts arrived at the following conclusion: "We now know exactly all of the elements contained in the human body, and therefore know what must be eaten for upbuilding—for replacement of used-up cells and for producing vitality, efficiency, strength and heat."

You were taught in former lessons why these "conclusions" are wrong and have produced the "protein" fad and later the "mineral-salt" fad and now the very latest fashion, i.e., the "raw-food" fad. Without knowledge of the "great unknown," their conclusions must be wrong. This great "unknown"— unknown to the chemical and medical experts—unknown to the average man and health seeker—unknown to the layman dietitian—unknown to the general dietetical systems now in vogue—and this "great unknown" is "O" in my formula: "V" equals "P" minus "O"—the waste, the mucus (acids and poisons), the OBSTRUCTIONS, or "O" in the sick and also in the average so-called "healthy human body."

In other words, if human nourishment could ever be figured by mathematical chemical formulas telling exactly what to eat, you will still be fooled by nature—just so long as any ideal food is mixed with, and put into, this waste of mucus and acids already in the human system through years of wrong living. Nature confuses you—so long as you fail to recognize her facts and her truths—but nature herself is not fooled. To the average layman, raw food reacts more or less mysteriously—as long as it is mixed with your own mucus, as long as it stirs up mucus and its toxemias in the unclean diseased body and eliminates these poisons. All laymen and experts covering the entire dietetical movement up to the present time are puzzled, confused, ignorant, and still in complete darkness of the fact that, in general, the average man first becomes worse (sometimes developing boils and all kinds of sores) [when he] starts what he believes is a correct and best diet—living on a radical fruit, mucusless or raw-food diet.

"Tell me what to eat," wails the sick, "I want a daily menu for my special disease" (like a drug prescription), and he then considers that as all- sufficient. When the elimination sets in, he says, "These foods don't agree with me," instead of recognizing that the transition diet has already started in a moderate way to dissolve and to eliminate the old waste in the body—with some disturbance, of course. You must make them realize the necessity of putting up with this temporary inconvenience and consider themselves fortunate indeed to be able to continue with their daily work instead of undergoing an operation, which would mean months in a hospital. The foods agree with them, but they do not agree with the foods.

Now you may understand why and in what manner I differ from all others. The "*Mucusless Diet Healing System*" is a system in which every change in diet has certain duties to perform—

as a diet of healing to be applied systematically according to the condition of the sick.[26]

***

Above, I have isolated one of the fundamental reasons why many have misunderstood or resisted Ehret's work. His proposition challenges the very foundation of Western dietetic theory, which has been taken up by most modern naturopathic modalities including raw foodism. With this said, it may be observed that the ultimate conclusion of Ehret's transitional "healing system" is mucus-free fruits and green-leaf vegetables (mucus-forming fruits like avocado would not be on the list). A mono-diet of fruit is yet a higher goal. This is one reason why Ehret is sometimes viewed specifically as a raw foodist or fruitarian. The logical conclusion of the *Mucusless Diet* is a mono-fruit diet or fruit and green leaves. Further, the implications of V=P-O even suggest a modality beyond eating. In fact, I've said before that I know of no other writer that goes beyond Ehret, as I have not yet heard any others deal with V=P-O.

With all of this said, Ehret's systematic method can and has been used by people of all walks of life to achieve various levels of health. People who aspire to be vegans, raw foodists, or fruitarians could use Ehret's methods to slowly and permanently transition to these levels of being. Above, I hoped to shed a bit of light on the issue of raw foodism from Ehret's perspective. I know that many of you may have learned of Ehret through the teachings of progressive natural healers and dietitians. In fact, many of the most famous modern gurus come directly or indirectly out of Ehret. However, most have adopted modern, "Western" explanations of nutrition and reference Ehret only for his contributions to fasting and experimentation with fruit diet. Yet, my proposition is that we take a closer look at Ehret's work and consider health from his perspective: V=P-O.

Peace, Love, and Breath!!!

-Prof. Spira

---

26. Ehret, Arnold, Prof. *Arnold Ehret's Mucusless Diet Healing System* (Los Angeles: Ehret Literature Pub. Co., 1924).

132

Fasting, Fatigue, and Weakness

Originally posted on the Arnold Ehret Facebook Page, c. 2009

Why is it that I get tired and weak whenever I try to fast? Also, why does the transition take so long?

> Fatigue is in the first place a reduction of strength by too much digestion work; secondly, a clogging up of the heated and consequently narrowed-down blood vessels; and thirdly, a self- and re-poisoning through the excretion of mucus during the motion.[27]

Here I would ask: What are the implications of Vitality = Power - Obstruction? Above, Ehret is speaking of different forms of fatigue, but the principle of V = P - O helps to explain them all. In the first case, most of the world's eaters need to sleep anywhere from 4 to 12 hours every 24 hours. In my view, sleep is essentially a "forced fast,"[28] where certain bodily faculties are shut down so that 1) eating is stopped, 2) the body can recuperate from being overstimulated from eating, and 3) waste materials (pus and mucus) can be prepared for excretion or, in the case of bodily constipation, assimilated into the tissue system of the organism. In the second case, when one restricts mucus-forming foods and/or the amount of food taken into the body, the body begins to go through a healing process. Pus and mucus that have been assimilated into the body after generations of mucus eating then begin to be brought to the surface for elimination. This material then obstructs the blood flow, creating understimulation. Further, the toxic, loosened waste enters the bloodstream to be eliminated, resulting in "re-poisoning." Here, as the blood becomes obstructed with latent waste materials, weakness sets in. Depending on the degree of toxicity, weakness is combined with feeling horrible.

To put the above into perspective I offer the following narratives:

> Brian, who is 4 years old, is in the living room of his house alone. In his hand he has a water gun. For some reason, he is urged to shoot water onto the electrical outlet that the television is plugged into. As he does this, his mother comes in

---

27. Ehret, Arnold, *Rational Fasting for Physical, Mental, and Spiritual Rejuvenation* (Los Angeles: Ehret Literature Pub., 1926), 25.

28. See page 286 for definition of "forced fast."

and sees him. She immediately takes the gun from him and scolds him. Although he begins to cry, he is aware that what he did is unfavorable to his mother. Consequently, he knew why he was scolded. Cause and effect: because he squirted the electrical socket with water, he was then scolded by his mother.

Tom, who is now also 4 years old, accidentally broke an antique lamp when he was 1 year old. He was learning to walk, fell, and knocked over a tall, skinny lamp. At the time, his mother acted as if nothing had happened. Three years later, Tom was sitting on the couch watching Saturday morning cartoons and his mother came in furious. She screamed at him and slapped him across the face. Tom began to cry. He was confused and did not know why his mother was so angry with him. After one last slap across the face, his mother storms out of the room. As Tom sits crying, he tries to figure out what he did wrong. What he did not realize was that his mother was furious at him for breaking the antique lamp, an event that he is not even aware that he did.

When it comes to physiological illness and elimination, many of us are in Tom's position. We must pay for having broken universal laws, but we do not make a connection between our past indiscretions and the pain and suffering that we are going through in the present moment. In the case of fatigue, we have been eating poisons that have kept us so high for so long, the process of coming down is much more horrendous than the process of getting off heroin or meth. We must eliminate the wrongdoing of generations of mucus poisoning. Thus, a lifetime of transition is in order. One question to consider is, How far back in your bloodline must you go before you meet your fruitarian ancestors? What is your physiological karma?[29] It must be understood that the uneliminated, assimilated wastes of any organism are passed onto the next generation. Consequently, we must suffer the effects of wrong eating from our ancestral bloodline as we eliminate waste. Weakness and fatigue are Mother Nature's punishment for our wrong living. But, since we have been running from her, by the time we get punished we have forgotten what we have done wrong. Now, equipped with knowing that eating pus and mucus is wrong, like jumping off of a building is wrong, we can understand the nature of our eliminations better.

29. See page 288 for definition of "physiological karma."

134

When I fast, I usually go through several days of feeling awful. I'm blowing my nose, moping around, feeling weak and tired. By the seventh or eighth day, I feel the warm embrace of Mother Nature. It is like an eternal hug. Of course, there are ups and downs within the course of the fast, but the warm hug is always felt. When I begin eating again, the hug becomes much harder to feel. The more I eat, the more disconnected I become.

Baptism: (from Essene Gospel of Peace, Book One)

And Jesus said: "After the angel of air, seek the angel of water. Put off your shoes and your clothing and suffer the angel of water to embrace all your body. Cast yourselves wholly into his enfolding arms, and as often as you move the air with your breath, move with your body the water also. I tell you truly, the angel of water shall cast out of your body all uncleanesses which defiled it without and within. And all unclean and evil-smelling things shall flow out of you, even as the uncleannesses of garments washed in water flow away and are lost in the stream of the river. I tell you truly, holy is the angel of water who cleanses all that is unclean and makes all evil-smelling things of a sweet odor. No man may come before the face of God whom the angel of water lets not pass. In very truth, all must be born again of water and of truth, for your body bathes in the river of earthly life, and your spirit bathes in the river of life everlasting. For you receive your blood from our Earthly Mother and the truth from our Heavenly Father.

"Think not that it is sufficient that the angel of water embrace you outwards only. I tell you truly, the uncleanness within is greater by much than the uncleanness without. And he who cleanses himself without, but within remains unclean, is like to tombs that outward are painted fair, but are within full of all manner of horrible uncleannesses and abominations. So I tell you truly, suffer the angel of water to baptize you also within, that you may become free from all your past sins, and that within likewise you may become as pure as the river's foam sporting in the sunlight.

"Think not that it is sufficient that the angel of water embrace you outwards only. I tell you truly, the uncleanness within is greater by much than the uncleanness without. And he who

135

cleanses himself without, but within remains unclean, is like to tombs that outwards are painted fair, but are within full of all manner of horrible uncleannesses and abominations. So I tell you truly, suffer the angel of water to baptize you also within, that you may become free from all your past sins, and that within likewise you may become as pure as the river's foam sporting in the sunlight.

"Seek, therefore, a large trailing gourd, having a stalk the length of a man; take out its innards and fill it with water from the river which the sun has warmed. Hang it upon the branch of a tree, and kneel upon the ground before the angel of water, and suffer the end of the stalk of the trailing gourd to enter your hinder parts, that the water may flow through all your bowels. Afterwards rest kneeling on the ground before the angel of water and pray to the living God that He will forgive you all your past sins, and pray the angel of water that he will free your body from every uncleanness and disease. Then let the water run out from your body, that it may carry away from within it all the unclean and evil-smelling things of Satan. And you shall see with your eyes and smell with your nose all the abominations and uncleanness which defiled the temple of your body; even all the sins which abode in your body, tormenting you with all manner of pains. I tell you truly, baptism with water frees you from all of these. Renew your baptizing with water on every day of your fast, till the day when you see that the water which flows out of you is as pure as the river's foam. Then betake your body to the coursing river, and there in the arms of the angel of water render thanks to the living God that He has freed you from your sins. And this holy baptizing by the angel of water is rebirth unto the new life. For your eyes shall henceforth see, and your ears shall hear. Sin no more, therefore, after your baptism, that the angels of air and of water may eternally abide in you and serve you ever more.

"And if afterward there remain within you aught of your past sins and uncleannesses, seek the angel of sunlight. Put off your shoes and your clothing and suffer the angel of sunlight to embrace all your body. Then breathe long and deeply, that the angel of sunlight may be brought within you. And the angel of sunlight shall cast out of your body all evil-smelling and

136

unclean things which defiled it without and within. And all unclean and evil-smelling things shall rise from you, even as the darkness of night fades before the brightness of the rising sun. For I tell you truly, holy is the angel of sunlight who cleans out all uncleannesses and makes all evil-smelling things of a sweet odor. None may come before the face of God, whom the angel of sunlight lets not pass. Truly, all must be born again of sun and of truth, for your body basks in the sunlight of the Earthly Mother, and your spirit basks in the sunlight of the truth of the Heavenly Father." (Edmond Bordeaux Szekely (1905–1979), trans. *Essene Gospel of Peace: Book One,* [accessed from www.essene.com/GospelOfPeace/peace1.html])

This excerpt is from the *Essene Gospel of Peace* translated by Edmond Bordeaux Szekely (1905–1979). There is a fair amount of controversy surrounding this text and the nature of its authenticity. Some believe that the healing abilities of Jesus are due in part to his knowledge of fruitarianism and fasting as the omnipotent healing modalities for humankind. There are a handful of books that offer fruitarian versions of other biblical characters, such as *The Essene Gospel of John,* which portrays John the Baptist as a fruitarian. Some people believe that the writings were constructed by Szekely and raw-food activist Johnny Lovewisdom to promote fruitarian consciousness. Others say that much of the breathairean and fruitarian consciousness that was found in original versions of ancient theological texts were suppressed or eliminated during Constantine's assemblage of the Bible. I do not know the true nature of their origins, nor do I feel it to be particularly important. I view the work as a great piece of literature that does allude to universal healing laws—one of the few to do so this explicitly. With that said, clues that point toward human's fundamental fruitarian nature may still be found in modern bibles, such as Genesis 1:29:

> Then God said, "Behold, I have given you every plant yielding seed that is on the surface of all the earth, and every tree which has fruit yielding seed; it shall be food for you. (New American Standard Bible 1995)

All in all, lemon enemas have been important to me. As our body loosens and attempts to throw off waste, we must do all that we can to help. I'm reminded of the chicken embryo experiment, where embryos were kept alive for many years. This was possible because the waste that they excreted was eliminated every day. After about 26 years, one day was missed of cleaning the waste out and the embryos died. It was proposed that the embryos could have survived indefinitely if the waste was continually eliminated. What is the level of health that we could attain if we were to consistently eliminate the waste that our body throws off?

Peace, Love, and Breath!

-Prof. Spira

Prof. Spira on Dry Fasting and the Cyclical Nature of the Transition

The following was initially written in response to several questions that I received about dry fasting. Recently, some dry- and water-fasting retreats/clinics have received increased public attention, and below I share some of my thoughts on the subject.

By Prof. Spira
9/23/2012

Dry fasting is certainly at the top of the mountain. But it is dangerous to do without having transitioned for a while. Arnold Ehret once loosely defined fasting as any restriction of food or liquid intake. Ultimately, fasting is a relative proposition. What fasting is for my body may not be the same for someone else's body. And this can even shift depending on the changes in your own physiology. To determine what fasting regimen is right for you, it is essential to understand various dynamics of your own body. What is the amount of uneliminated waste in your bowels? Do you have a uric (acid) lean body type, or a fatty (mucus) body type? Uric acid types are those that are often said to have "high metabolisms" and can seemingly eat a lot and not get fat. The misconception is that this person is healthier than an overweight person. This is often not the case, as their body just handles mucus and pus differently than fatty (mucus) types.

Knowing that I am a mucus-type greatly informs how I approach the transition diet and the proposition of fasting on various levels. (See Arnold Ehret's *Mucusless Diet Healing System* for more on physiological types.) There is a world of experiences from dry to water fasting; a world between dry and fruit-juice fasting; light years between achieving such fasts while doing regular enemas; worlds between fruit-juice and fruit/vegetable-juice fasting; a galaxy between cooked-juice (store-bought juice) and fresh, raw-juice fasting; a universe between juice fasting and (mucus-free) fresh-fruit fasting (I now have to make the distinction of mucus-free fruit, since many folks eat and view the fatty/mucus-forming ones as fruits fit for fasting); an omniverse between eating a raw, mucusless diet and a cooked, mucus-lean one; and, of course, there is a multi-dimensional omniversal black hole between a plant-based, mucus-lean reality and the standard pus-and-mucus existence. And each of these realities can be considerably different depending upon how long and how well you have transitioned toward a cleansing diet. Doing a dry fast after 40 years of mucusless

139

transition is much different than doing one after a year of eating raw or vegan.

Although we might be tempted to view healing as a linear progression, I encourage you to consider it from multiple perspectives. It may be advantageous to view this as a continuum rather than a strict line. A continuum may be defined as a sequence in which adjacent elements are not perceptibly different from each other, although the extremes are quite distinct. Thus, I am referring to a continuum—or cycle—of physiological realities. And each reality corresponds with a field of consciousness. My personal goal is to eliminate all of my physiological and emotional karma and ultimately emancipate myself from continually having to experience the lower end of this cycle.

With that said, I have given only a brief overview of what some would call the "physical" side of things. How are these levels of fasting affected by practices in the science of breath and meditation? What if instead of always breathing 60 times a minute, we slowed it down to 30 or less (consider how fast a dog breaths and how short their lives are)? How does sunbathing affect the various levels of fasting? Regular colon irrigation? Music-making? Astral travels, herbs, healing massage, etc.? Each one of these are profound realities in themselves, but when combined with various levels of fasting, unexplored vistas of experience and fields of consciousness open up.

I mention this to offer a perspective on the dynamics and sophistication involved in considering the various levels of fasting. Yet, many people are not aware of this and feel compelled to go from one end of the spectrum to the other with little or no transition. On one hand, progressive sanitariums and fasting retreats can be very beneficial. (Brother Air and I plan to open a *Mucusless Diet* sanitarium and fasting retreat in the future.) On the other hand, most practitioners do not leave these retreats equipped to transform the short-term successes that might be gained into a long-term reality. As soon as everyone goes home and partially heals their ailments, many relapse into old habits when they least expect it. Short-term success can be gained; but without the tools and intentions to begin mastering the physiological continuum, relapse is almost inevitable.

As I mention above, fasting is relative. When Brother Air—who has practiced the *Mucusless Diet* for over 30 years—dry fasts, it is very different from when others health seekers do it. Having removed the obstructions from the cells of his body, he is ready to dry fast and truly

140

benefit from it on a long-term basis. I think his longest stint was over 40 days dry, and he often does shorter ones regularly. It is just not a big deal for him at this point. In fact, he has been shifting between dry and juice fasting for the past couple of months and endeavors to do another extended fast.

I've done two 14-day dry fasts, one followed by months of fruit-juice fasting. The first one occurred early on my journey as I was eliminating quarts of mucus from my body. The second one was last year. After a couple days, I no longer was thirsty and things felt wonderful. The experience was incredible and best illustrated by the music I made at those times. Yet, my fasting usually comes about through instinct. I've spent a great deal of my time mentally preparing myself to "let go" and allow my body to do its thing (see my blog post on Intuition vs. Intellect in the Art of the Transition Pt 1: http://www.mucusfreelife.com/art-transition-diet-mucusless/).

This is different than people who use their mind to plan out a specific fast with a predetermined length of time. For me, it is best to eliminate the mind chatter so that I can let my body lead the way. Sometimes my body seems to move faster than my mind can follow, so I make an effort to free my mind of obstruction. This led me to critically analyze many of our socially conditioned beliefs, particularly in the area of human dietetics. I spent a lot of time researching the origins of Western dietetic thought. Why do I believe in a protein theory developed in 1830 by people doing sadistic experiments on dogs? Why has no one even let me know that it is merely a theory (a bad one at that)? Where did modern nutritional concepts come from? By critically interrogating the origins of such concepts, I began to truly free my mind of such nonsensical drivel (I challenge anyone to look into the history of these theories and not be blown away by how weak and problematic they are). Consequently—in the midst of a fast—conditioned, fear-based mind-chatter like, "Wow, I haven't eaten in a couple months so I better break it and get some protein" did not occur.

I find such concepts as good/bad bacteria, protein, B-12, vitamins, and the like to be very problematic and, at least for me, un-useful. We need no probiotics or other kinds of supplementation. Yet, our Western conditioning has programmed us to feel as if we always need to take something. Probiotics, B-12, vitamins, etc., all are mental and, if consumed, physical obstructions. I like what naturopath Dr. Robert Morse had to say about about vitamins and B-12 in a video: "I just don't

141

go there, and I don't think any animal does [either]." Hanging onto such theories can hold us back from physiological liberation.

Fasting is the omnipotent healing force for animal life. Yet, there are levels within levels, upon levels, of fasting—and it is different for each physical body (not to mention astral bodies). My proposition is to start where you are and slowly and safely transition toward higher levels. Don't feel as if you need to do long fasts or dry fasts. Strive to do Rational Fasts based upon your own body. A lot of people play basketball, but few people think that they should be able to play like Michael Jordan without serious practice and long-term dedication. Yet, in dietetics, health seekers often feel as if they should be able to skip over worlds of experience without any practice. Dry fasting is a worthy goal, but something to work toward through long-term practice of the mucusless diet. Most people are far too obstructed with mucus, pus, and acids for a dry fast to be very beneficial. The purpose of liquid or solid food is to help eliminate waste that has been loosened by a period of fasting. But, after years of practice, dry fasting becomes natural.

One aspect of healing and fasting which is often underdiscussed is the relationship between healing and emotional eliminations. As we live out and evolve our physiological karma, all corners of our reality, those seen and unseen, evolve. On the subject of emotional development and elimination, I pour my message and feelings into my art and writings. I'm a jazz musician and it was my musical journey that led me to the work of Arnold Ehret and the mucusless diet. When I make music, I can express joy, laughter, sadness, rage, disappointment, peace, love, and/or breath. I feel the best when I am creating. When I let go and allow the art to flow—I don't even think about eating. Making music has always played a large role in the success of my longer fasts. I sustain myself with music. Channeling sound and vibration from the Universe is so much easier and more fulfilling while I'm fasting. The cleaner and more empty I become, the more music I am filled with. And making music with others who are also fasting is one of the most incredible experiences! Wise men and women often say that we must be empty—an optimally clean body, which simultaneously absorbs and emits energy while reflecting none, or as Arnold Ehret simply put it, Vitality = Power − Obstruction!—in order to be filled with the omnipotent spirit of the Universe.

Peace, Love, and Breath!

Prof. Spira

Chapter 5—The Wader Family Consultations

Introduction

You read my first interactions with the Tim and Samantha Wader from the Ehret Club Forum in the first chapter. As their questions became more personal, I offered to consult with them via email. Below are some of our conversations.

Further Exploring the B-12 Myth

Email from Wader on December 25, 2005 3:53 PM

Hi Spira!

We would love to hear more of your thoughts about B-12. Spira, our family truly thanks you for your assistance and your consideration.

Have a wonderful day!

Sincerely,

-Tim and Samantha

Spira's Response:

Email from Professor Spira on Monday, December 26, 2005 11:07 AM

Greetings,

It is wonderful to hear about your family's progress on the *Mucusless Diet Healing System* and great to communicate with people who are really serious about their health. Here are several additional thoughts about the B-12 myth:

Whenever we are provoked by the erroneous concepts that we have been programmed to respect since childhood, we must have courage in the unknown. Simple logic will always save the day. I know plenty of people who were pus-and-mucus eaters that have suffered and died from disease, but I do not know anybody who died eating only fruits and green, leafy vegetables (mucusless foods). Since we already know what is at the end of the mucus path, it makes sense to explore the unknown. I find it essential to interrogate the historical origins of these erroneous medical and dietetic theories. Who created the protein myth and when? Who coined the term *vitamin* and why? What kind of diet did these elusive founding fathers of Western medical science have, and how did it affect the nature of their investigations? Consider the historical origin of the B-12 theory that I eluded to earlier:

> B-12 deficiency is the cause of several forms of anemia. The treatment for this disease was first devised by William Murphy, who bled dogs to make them anemic and then fed them various substances to see what (if anything) would make them healthy again. He discovered that ingesting large amounts of liver seemed to cure the disease. George Minot and George Whipple then set about to chemically isolate the curative substance and ultimately were able to isolate Vitamin B-12 from the liver. For this, all three shared the 1934 Nobel Prize in Medicine. ("B-12 History," Wikipedia: accessed 2005)

Thus, through a sadistic experiment on a dog (not a human), Murphy reasoned that pus (rotting flesh) helped to save an anemic dog from certain death. Twisted and absurd! Unfortunately, far too many of the origin stories that form our dietetic and medical mythology derive from sordid scenarios such as this one.

So if Vitamin B-12 does not exist, what do medical doctors measure in a B-12 blood test?

Short answer, they (doctors) can't see the forest for the trees and don't know what they are looking at. Long answer: a chemist might say "cyanocobalamin," merely the name invented for a particular chemical structure found in the body. Since the days of alchemy, humans have had a fascination with extracting, isolating, naming, and examining chemical components. This proved to be useful when extracting metals from ore, making pigment for paints and make-up, or concocting questionable medicinal potions that suppress symptoms of elimination. However, it must be understood that the foundation on which Western

144

physiology and medical science is built is egregiously erroneous. Based on their own omnivorous diets, early researchers assumed that humans needed to eat dead animal flesh, etc. Given the historical context surrounding the eating habits of these early investigators, it is easy to see why the foundation of their physiological inquiry is so flawed. They failed to consider the proposition that humans are a tropical, frugivorous species, and that the foundation of human illness is constipation/obstruction derived from unnatural food substances. This resulted in a problematic "additive paradigm" to emerge, whereby the intake of (wrong) foods for fuel became the emphasis. In the *Mucusless Diet Healing System*, Prof. Arnold Ehret explains that

> Metabolism, or the "science of change of matter," is the most absurd and the most dangerous doctrine-teaching ever imposed on mankind. It is the father of the wrong cell theory and of that most erroneous albumen theory, which latter theory will kill and stamp out the entire civilized Western world if its following is not stopped.[30]

The French medical term *anemia* derives from the Greek "anaimia," which means "lack of blood" or "bloodless." In 1822, a Scottish doctor wrote a report on the "History of a Case of Anemia," which is the name eventually given to this condition of cellular constipation. Interestingly, the Scottish doctor theorized that the illness derived from digestion or absorption issues. It was only 40 years ago that American doctors proposed that the problem was associated with their problematic concept of nutrition. I do not deny the existence of particular kinds of chemical structures that may be observed in the body with sophisticated modern tools. The problem is that what these chemicals do and how they operate are misunderstood.

In medicine, flawed theories are built upon older flawed theories, which results in total confusion. It is still believed by many that humans need to eat rotting carcasses to obtain some kind of nutrition. And if not enough is eaten, it must be supplemented by chemical isolates (poisons) or with an increase of certain fruits/vegetables. This medieval thinking is still the foundation of Western dietetic thought. Yet, what cow drinks milk to produce milk or eats other cows to produce beef? What 600-

---

30. Ehret, Arnold, *Arnold Ehret's Mucusless Diet Healing System: A Complete Course for Those Who Desire to Learn How to Control Their Health* (Dobbs Ferry, NY: Ehret Literature), 64.

pound gorilla needs B-12 supplements or shots (unless unfortunate enough to be imprisoned by humans)? My proposition is that such reasoning of medical science is greatly flawed, and it is necessary to dispense with many of these commonly held notions.

In a world where mucus and pus eating runs rampant, and clueless medical doctors are unquestionably respected like clergymen, the fear of not getting enough "nutrition" still exists. A new physiological paradigm based upon the principles of Ehret's "New Physiology" must be explored and further realized. With this said, the SYMPTOMS associated with our modern concept of "deficiency" are real, although the explanation for why they occur is fallacious. Given that constipation is the foundation of human illness, it must be understood that such experiences derive from a condition of cellular constipation. Removing this waste and regenerating on the cellular level may only be done perfectly and permanently through the long-term practice of the *Mucusless Diet Healing System.*

Peace, Love, and Breath!

-Prof. Spira

Eating Nuts and the Worldwide Mucusless Movement

Email from Professor Spira on Monday, December 26, 2005 12:11 PM

Greetings!

In regard to your questions about nuts, I used things that worked for Brother Air. His main nut menus consisted of usually peanuts and cashews mixed always with raisins. He also advocates peanut butter and jelly on wheat toast for the days when mucus cravings are high. For me, analyzing the type of nut is not all that important, since it is all going to be eliminated eventually. I would recommend trying to find nuts that digest and eliminate well for you. Depending on your individual physiology, you will find certain kinds of foods effective and/or ineffective. In fact, nuts are very hard for me to eat now; they make me feel dreadful. I did not plan on eliminating nuts out of my diet so soon, but my body just does not want to have anything to do with them. My craving for nuts may eventually come back, but they are inedible right now. But the goal is to get our bodies so clean that it is impossible for us to eat the wrong foods. As for the sugars, I stick with the sweeteners that Ehret suggests, including *real* brown sugar (not white sugar dyed brown) and honey. Ehret spends a substantial amount of time talking about the ways in which sugar, namely fruit sugar, breaks down to a non-sticky substance in the body, and that most fruits break down to form a mucusless syrup. The key to the formation of mucus in the body is constipation. If you are doing enemas every day, whatever is going in is going to keep moving.

In regards to the conventions and expos about the diet, you are actually witnessing the beginning of a worldwide movement where the *Mucusless Diet Healing System* is introduced to the masses by people who live it. For the past 30 years, the practitioners in Cincinnati, OH have stayed relatively quiet and to themselves. Without eating pus and mucus, they did not have the stimulation or the resources to try to educate the world. They had to live the diet in a time when it seemed that nobody wanted to be bothered with it. Over the past couple of years, there has been a surge in the interest in the diet, and the amount of serious practitioners in this camp has increased faster than it ever has before. When I started the diet, I did not think that the world was ready to deal with it yet, and I figured that I would quietly practice the diet like my predecessors—maybe even spend some years living secluded in the woods fasting and meditating. However, recent events that happened in my life and around our community, as well as cultural shifts, indicated to me that it is time for a major push. The technology is to the point where with the click of a mouse, millions of peoples' consciousnesses can be raised. I've decided to dedicate my life to developing an organization that will inform the world about the *Mucusless Diet Healing System* and where it has been taken. My goal is to eventually put on big seminars and conventions where people can come and receive some information that they can really use. After this, we will open a sanitarium, and so on. Once the website is operational, we will be ready to start serious promotion. It is great to have supporters like you who reaffirm to me that it is the proper time for the *Mucusless Diet* to be revealed.

I will talk to you soon.

Peace, Love, and Breath!

-Prof. Spira

Email from the Wader Family on Monday, December 26, 2005 12:11 PM

Hi Spira!

We have been eating almonds, Brazil nuts, walnuts, and hazelnuts, usually mixed with raisins, figs, or dates. The reason for those choices is, from our research, much of the information available to us has shown those types of nuts to be closer to neutral in the acidic/alkaline tables. Hopefully, we are correct in that approach. Is there a particular reason why Brother Air always mixes them with raisins though? When it comes to the wheat toast, is that a home-prepared wheat bread or a certain store-bought brand made well enough for intake? In our research here, it seems that many of the offers of wheat bread in the stores, even health food co-ops, contain some ingredients which didn't feel all that comfortable to us, but then I remember reading how Arnold explained when your breads are very well toasted, they are made better/safer for eating.

I can hardly wait to be clean enough to be able to reject foods which are bad for me. It has already happened with popcorn for me. Even the smell of it causes me to have to leave the room. Incredible to me, as that was at one time a most favorite snack, especially when the family gathers for watching a movie. Now, we do still watch movies, but we spend a lot of time as a family discussing the diet and playing mind-stimulating, strategic board games and eating proper snacks—only when we actually feel the need to snack, that is, but not as a habit.

Your words written about progressing on a global scale to inform the world and drop the informational bomb truly caused a positive electrical impulse in our souls. Powerful! We were so immensely thrilled and excited to read it!

I don't believe there is a proper enough way to say, with absolute sincerity, Thank You!

Have a most perfect day and we look forward to talking with you again soon!

With all sincerity, God Bless,

-Tim and Samantha

Losing Weight and Physiological Karma

Email sent by the Wader Family on Wednesday, December 28, 2005 8:51 AM

Hi Spira!

We hope your week is going very well! We were wondering about weight. I believe I mentioned that our son was on the diet originally for about 3 weeks, then fell of the diet for about a week as he saw our daughter give up pretty quickly. Then, after that week, he felt the consequences of his decision in his body and went back on the diet. Our son is going to be 17 in February and our daughter is 14. Well, he is now starting his third week of restarting the diet and he has lost 6 pounds in the past week. He is concerned that he is losing too much, too fast. I've lost almost 40 pounds myself since beginning the diet on October 29th, but seem to have stabilized at around 155 pounds or so. In your and your colleagues' experiences, would this be considered losing too much weight too fast? If so, what is the best approach to correcting that?

Also, my wife, who is going on I believe it is her sixth to seventh week of the diet, said she has lost hardly any weight at all. She is wondering if something may be wrong in what she is doing (there doesn't really appear to be), as everyone else is losing weight so fast. She was a very heavy goat milk, yogurt, protein mix, vitamin/supplement taker, yet snacked a lot throughout the day (usually cookies, chips, crackers, etc.) because she is hypoglycemic. She also seems to be having a more difficult time—feeling bad, hurting, and tired—during the transition than we are. Would there be some reason to explain to her why she is not losing as much and suffering so much more? Have you and your colleagues found that it is more difficult or slower for women to reach their optimum weight level than men or have a more difficult time during the transition?

Thank you Spira! Have an incredible day!

Sincerely,

-Tim, Samantha, and Little Joey

Email Sent by Professor Spira on Thursday, December 29, 2005 11:18 AM

Greetings!

Physiologically speaking, you must understand that once the body starts going down the road of cleansing, it is making a 180-degree turn from its former direction. The filth in the body will do everything it can to try and convince you to get away from the *Mucusless Diet Healing System*. Psychological warfare is some of the most intensive weaponry that your body will use against you. This is where the subject of weight comes in. We are programmed by cultural norms to be so concerned with weight. In fact, it is generally accepted that fat and skinny people are unhealthy, while thicker, muscle-bound people are healthy. Skinny people who can eat morbid amounts of food and not get any bigger are also put on a pedestal. Everything in our culture is in an inverted position.

Physiological Types—We understand that the skinny patient who has a great "metabolism" in actuality is a uric-acid type, where the mucus they eat is burned by the toxic waste in their bodies. Obese people are usually mucus types, and their bodies endeavor to tuck the uneliminated waste into the tissue system away from the heart and lungs. Depending on what type of physiology you currently are will tell you how much weight you will lose and what type of transition your body needs. (Let me know what physiology type you believe you and your family are so that I can better assess your individual concerns). When I met Brother Air ,I was a 280-pound mucus type. When we started talking about the diet, we never even talked about weight; all of the emphasis was placed on the diet, with the knowledge that the weight is eventually going to be whatever it is supposed to be. It is easier said than done because of the psychological battles that we will face. As I lost weight, I traveled through what I call my perfect American size. I went from a 40-inch waist to a 36 at about 210 pounds, my muscles were really defined, and I felt good. People (especially females) were attracted to me like never before. I enjoyed this period, but I knew that I could not get attached to it and that I would need to move forward when my physiology was ready. My next stop was a 33-inch waist. It was basically the "male model" size. I was still shaving, but I had stopped cutting my hair. At this point, the thrill was gone from surprising old friends with my transformation. Now, when I see old football buddies and people who used to look up to me as a muscle-bound football player, they would give me this look of fear. They could not understand why I would want to lose so much weight. I, of course, would tell them that I did not try to lose this weight but it just happened as a result of changing my diet.

Now, if anything can be drawn from my story, understand that as you go through the diet, the way you see the world will change. Do not let the words from ignorant outsiders deter you from following the path. Misery loves company, and the people around you will do everything they can to lure you back to a life of pain and suffering.

Losing a nice amount of weight early on is common. If transitional menus, fasting, and enemas are systematically put together, old weight from the 32 feet of impacted intestines will start being eliminated, immediately lightening your load. In the case of your son, let me know a little about what he is eating on and off the diet. Both of your children have a wonderful opportunity to start the transition at such a young age. In fact, the psychological struggles may often seem harder than the physiological.

As Ehret says, at some points during the elimination the patient will look horrible, will get really thin, and will suffer some heavy emotional disturbances. In fact, before my long fast, I was looking pretty bad and then I actually gained weight during the fast. We must retrain our soiled perceptions to accept our natural, skinny, healthy appearances.

Physiological Karma—Everybody possesses what I call physiological karma. It is what each individual must go through to pay reparations for not only what they have done to themselves, but the compounded physiological karma from their parents, grandparents, and so forth. This means that some individuals will suffer from being very tired and weak, while others will suffer intense emotional instability [I'm raising my hand], and some will find it hard to deal with the psychological acceptance of the *Mucusless Diet Healing System* and all of the responsibilities that come with it. You must analyze your strengths and weaknesses in order to better understand why you are the way you are. I find that I am advanced in the psychological and physiological areas but that my cross to bear is an emotional one. Another individual I know can deal with the physiological but the psychological is her rough spot. Understanding your karma will not magically eliminate your problems, but it will help you pay your reparations thankfully. We know that the eating of improper foods is the reason for any and all of these problems, so the most important thing is to control what we put in our mouths by any *rational* means necessary!

In the case of your wife, she will have to be aware of her eliminations due to the heavy vitamin/chemical intake. I took toxic prescription medications since I was 7 years old and have a great deal of

152

old chemicals in my tissue system. As I'm going through elimination, I can feel—usually in my heart area—the difference between chemical eliminations and mucus eliminations. I will have heart palpitations and suffer anxiety. It is important that these old chemicals not all hit the bloodstream at once. I've found the best foods to use through this to be large amounts of steamed broccoli and big salads. You may be surprised at how toxic your eliminations are in these periods (the toxins would actually try to eat away at my skin on their way out of my body).

Regarding your question about pepper, I try to avoid pure pepper when I can. Most of the people in this camp use salt-free Mrs. Dash seasonings and a vinegar-free salad dressing named Annie's Organic Green Garlic Dressing. However, a better raw dressing can be made that is free of any preservatives or questionable oils. We identify salt and products that contain vinegar to be the most dangerous condiments to be avoided (as well as high fructose corn syrup). However, as Ehret says, at this stage of the transition, the condiments are not as important to focus on as the mucus-forming foods. If you focus on changing the foods, your taste buds will start rejecting harmful condiments. Sometimes I can just take a head of lettuce and eat it savoring the natural sugar in the leaves. Other times I have to cover it with onions and garlic. My cravings all depend on my current elimination.

Regarding nuts, Brother Air always told me that the kind of nut is not as important as mixing it with dried fruit. The nuts give you that mucus satisfaction, but without the raisins they are not going to eliminate very easily. The dried fruit helps your intestines eliminate the nuts. The type of bread that we use is the 100-percent-sprouted-wheat Ezekiel Bread found in the health food section (usually frozen). The key to the bread is toasting it very well, which helps destroy its sticky properties. At this point, try to eat these transitional mucuses only when you crave them, and eat them accompanied with the correct foods. They can also be of benefit when you go through older cravings for things that you know your body cannot handle anymore.

I encourage all of you to keep up the good work. Your physiological investment will definitely not go unrewarded. As you repay your debts, you will get closer and closer to superior health. Shrug off the naysayers and focus on your physiological goals.

Health Is Wealth!

-Prof. Spira

Physiological Details about the Wader Family

Email from the Wader Family on Thursday, December 29, 2005 11:18 a.m.

Hi Spira!

I must say that our family is deeply thankful for such a detailed reply. Finally, some answers that are real, true, and very well thought through. Thank you!! I will try to answer some of your questions and outline them by individual to let you know what we've done and where we are at:

Little Joey (our son)—We believe he is more the uric-acid type. He has always been on the thin side. He is about 6'2" and currently, as of last night, about 125.7 lbs. He started with the first 2-week menu of the diet, and then fell off the diet for about 1 to 1½ weeks. When he came off the diet, he really made up for it by eating things such as toasted cinnamon bagels with melted cheese and a slice of ham; cereal with milk; daily sandwiches with three slices of ham, a slice of cheese, mayo, lettuce, salt and pepper; Safeway brand Hostess-type packaged apple pies; pepperoni Hot Pockets; soda; ice cream; energy drinks; chocolate; tacos; Pringles; chips and salsa dip; cookies; microwave popcorn; cup of noodles; top ramen soups; chewy bars; pizza; hot dogs. So, as you can see, he really fell off there. He restarted the diet with a 2-day fast. He has been through the first 2 weeks of the transition menu and is now at the beginning of the second 2 weeks of the menu, eating for 3 days, and then fasting for 2 days. He is having difficulty with being hungry a lot, wanting to "munch"/snack, and is also suffering from a lot of skin breakouts: dry/red rashes, dermatitis, acne, etc.

My Wife—She believes she is more the mucus type. She gains weight more easily and in the past has had to work out and barely eat to lose it or keep it off. She also believes she has been in early menopause after she had her tubes burned. She suffers from many female issues: yeast, bladder infections, severe cramps, long menstruations, etc. for years. The diet so far is putting her through some very difficult pains all over and irritations/pain in respect to the female problems/areas. She is also hypoglycemic. She seems to be having the most difficult time, but she is deeply firm on never giving up on this diet, as after studying she has discovered the errors of her past ways.

154

She started the diet back on November 19, but sort of in her own way trying to speed things up. She fasted 2 days, ate for a couple, and then fasted for 5 days, not following the course very close. She was feeling awful. So, around the December 1, I had her restart and try to stay structured with Arnold's first 2-week menu, eat for 3 days, then fast for a day until the first 2 weeks were up. Then, start the second 2-week menu, eat for 3 days, fast for 2 days, etc., and build her way up. Only trouble is, she has stuck with the first 2-week menu since December 1 and has not come off that yet. She said that she is in fear of the fruit part of the diet because of her female issues, yeast and irritations/pain during urination, etc., so she has been eating mostly the salads/vegetables. I did convince her last night to make the move toward the second 2-week menu, eating for 3 days, fasting for 2, etc. and trying to remain structured, becoming more restricted as time progresses. She said that she just has to make it past her fear of the unknown because some of the methods she has used in the past for her yeast and female issues worked for her (she has stopped all of that now: goat milk, goat yogurts, goat proteins, vitamins, etc.) and break through the payback period of what she has done to her body in the past. She said she has lost 14 lbs. since November 19. I believe what is happening, too, is she is watching me and trying to compare, speed things up to catch up, etc.; but like Arnold said, each individual is their own case and you can't speed up the healing system.

She has been having pains in the heart area, so when she does, she breaks her fasts. She is also beginning to have blood veins break, especially in her fingers/hands, and she is noticing that she is now bruising very, very easily. She has been noticing some minor varicose veins going away in her legs, though. But, her absolute first main concern is her female area issues.

Myself—I am around 6'2". I have always been on the thin side, probably uric-acid type, up until the past few years. In my younger days, I had a 30- to 31-inch waist, sometimes 29. Over the past few years, I've gone up to around 190-205 pounds. I started the diet on October 29 at around 190 lbs and a tight 36-inch waist. I am now at a loose 34-inch waist and seemed to have settled for now at around 154-155 pounds. Also, over the past years, I loved my Bud Light. I have been off any alcohol for a while now. I also smoked since the seventh grade. Eleven years ago, I quit for about 8 years. I restarted about 3 years ago and plan on trying to quit in about 3 more days. I also love my coffee. I actually drink quite a bit of it, too much. I work the midnight shift, which I am trying to fix now and go to a day-shift schedule, but I believe that is what has me hooked on the coffee so bad. My sleep and pattern of sleep is not all that great, terrible in fact, especially on days off, unfortunately.

I have followed the diet religiously since the beginning. As of last night, I am now through the fourth 2-week menu, broke a 3-day fast, ate a nice salad, steamed broccoli (then fell asleep before a bowel movement or enema, and will begin your prior recommendation to me of what to eat starting today, along with a lemon.) I would eat 3 days, fast for 1 day (in the beginning), then 2 days and now 3-day fasts, trying to build up to 5 or more. I have trouble sometimes due to my schedule constraints; sleep schedules, etc. to do a *lemona* every day. Sometimes—often, actually—I unfortunately go until the third day without a bowel movement until the enemas. The greatest pains I feel are in the area of my spleen. They get pretty intense during the fasts.

We all are suffering from feeling pretty tired, sluggish, and fatigued but with myself, I feel that is mostly due to my schedule because for the 2 weeks prior to returning to work from the fibromyalgia/narcolepsy, I was feeling incredible.

I hope this helps let you know more of where we are at, along with the concerns and struggles we're having. All three of us are most definitely committed to the diet at this point. I know that my wife and I will never go back for sure. Our son does still deal a bit with the psychological influences, but he is holding pretty strong so far, as one of his best friends is also on the diet now with his own struggles of no parental support at all. Yet his friend is deeply committed to following the diet as best he can under those conditions. We are very proud of Little Joey for the efforts he is making.

Spira, running into you has indeed been a blessing for us and the assistance of you and your colleagues is truly, so very deeply, appreciated by our family. Thank you so very, very much with all sincerity! Please, as you talk with your colleagues, pass on our deepest gratitude to them as well.

With deep sincerity,

Tim, Samantha, and Little Joey

God Bless

Transitioning More Slowly

Sent by Professor Spira on Friday, December 30, 2005 11:18 AM

Greetings!

Overall, I believe that your family needs to transition a bit slower. Those that are able to do the recommended weekly program comfortably should go for it. But remember that these were the menus Ehret used for his patients in his sanitarium. In many cases, they would be near death and unable to eat anything except what was given to them. After a couple of months, they would be healed and go right back to their old habits. Your son's experience is something that can happen in a traumatic way down the line. There are so many stories of people who manage to go great lengths of time on cleansing diets, but a couple years down the road they would have a near-fatal fall when all of the old poisons come back to eliminate. These poisons must be eliminated from the beginning. This can be achieved with a slower transition. When you are pursuing the diet as a lifestyle, personal thought and intuitions must be taken into consideration. Learn to use Ehret's menus as a tool toward the goal of mucus elimination.

In Little Joey's case, I believe he just needs to go on an easier transition. As a uric-acid type, I would recommend that he not fast as often, but concentrate on using more vegetables. When I started the diet, I was too filthy and addicted to what I was eating to attempt Ehret's weekly programs. But I used them as a place I would like to eventually be. I had to figure out a way to transition into the transition. I started adding much more green to everything. Then, before I knew it, the old mucuses were gone and I was in another place. I believe that Little Joey needs to really be hitting menus like the steamed broccoli and cabbage. Also, if he is craving snacks, then he can go with it but remain consistent with the enemas. Just try to one-up yourself from whatever you crave. If you crave white potato chips, eat sweet potato chips; if you crave candy, eat nuts with raisins instead. He should not be suffering from such hunger. In the uncomfortable time, it is great to get in the habit of first doing an enema. If I crave something I know I do not need, I just make a deal with myself that if I still crave it after an enema, I will eat it. Usually, the enema turns my craving into an absurd thought. The key is still the enemas. Really study yourself. Watch the food going in and study it on the way out. When you start seeing 2-foot long strands of mucus floating in the toilet, you will know you are on the right track. And do not be hard on yourself. Everybody that I know who has practiced the diet has fallen back to some old foods again, in the beginning. The extreme case is Ehret, who after 2 years on fruit "experimented" with eating meat again. The key is changing one's physiology so that the mere thought of a pizza or a ham sandwich sends fear into your heart. A slow, comfortable transition is the key. Furthermore, from a semantic point of view, we would call all of what Little Joey went through part of his transition. Part of the transition is falling, getting beat up, and getting back up. When you get back up, you will be stronger.

With your wife, I would not be too concerned with her not moving around to many other menus. At this stage in the game, if you find a groove, it is good to *wear it out*. You will see a natural change. Use the menu as a guide and understand why it works. Study how Ehret sets up his weekly plan and you will see the systematic nature of his approach. In any equation of the diet, time is the variable factor. Strive to understand how the system works and your informed intuition will lead you down the right path. With the symptoms that your wife is having, I would not recommend fasting as much as I would recommend mucusless menus with raw and steamed vegetables. The chemicals from the years of supplements must be eliminated through the bloodstream and kidneys as opposed to the bowels. The vegetables will slow the elimination so that it is not too uncomfortable or dangerous.

In your case, it sounds like what you have done thus far has been a nice transition. However, I would implore you to adopt the daily lemon enema. For anybody that wants to maximize their potential on the diet, the lemon enema is a must. One thing about the people in this camp is that the diet comes first. Everything in our lives revolves around the diet. If I am going through an elimination, I stay at home in bed and I don't worry about school. I find that whenever somebody truly puts the diet first, all of the worldly things take care of themselves. I also would only do as much fasting as is comfortable. Realize that the first couple of years while on the diet, you are running on the old mucus in the body. Old stimulants that are being eliminated enable one to do long fasts in the beginning. So go for it, but be ready for long eating bouts down the road once the old stuff is eliminated. The key is to be on fruits and green-leaf vegetables during these bouts. For instance, Brother Air went through an entire year—after years of practicing the diet—where it was hard to even fast for a day. At this stage in the game, strive to be mucusless for long periods of time. The fasting will come out of this.

In regards to being tired, this will happen. Remember how Ehret said that when an individual starts a diet of healing they feel great; then the elimination starts happening and it's not as fun. One of the hardest things for people to do is to just sit still and let the body do its thing. We are stimulant driven. As Brother Air often says, our current existence is all about being high. We get up, run and eat mucus, a little coffee, run to work, go to the bar, run to Blockbuster, to the arcade, shakin' it at the dance club, etc. Take stimulants out of the equation. This chaotic kind of lifestyle will not exist anymore. A much slower, calmer, and more effective way of life will present itself. Think about it. We are coming down from the mother of all drugs, mucus. It is like coming down from being drunk or high. You start out high, then as you come down you feel horrible. After being normal for a while, you then feel better. So look at the big picture of the diet and compare. If someone drinks for 2 hours, it may take another 2 hours to come down, accompanied with the karmic suffering that comes with eliminating the poisons. If someone has eaten mucus for 20 years, how long will the fall be?[31] The time is the variable/unknown for such a question. The time is dependent on the individual's physiology, constitutional encumbrances, and application of the system. However, we have eaten mucus for so long that the coming-down process takes a long time. We must be mindful of the diet from the big picture and be patient as we come down from the original gateway drug—mucus.

Berg's Table

What is the usefulness of the Berg table, which Ehret features in the *Mucusless Diet*? The Berg table can be problematic and confusing for first-time readers. In fact, some Ehretists believe that future editions of the *Mucusless Diet* should omit or annotate the section. Ultimately, it must be taken with a grain of salt and considered more critically. Ehret says that "the majority of foods he [Berg] calls 'acid-forming' are what I call 'mucus-forming,' and what he calls 'acid-binding,' that is, non-acid food, is almost exactly what I call 'mucusless'."[32] The key phrases are "the majority" and "almost exactly." Then he explains that "the mere fact that some foods in the list are 'acid-binding' does not necessarily

---

31. For definition of "the fall," see page 285.

32. Ehret, *MDHS* 1994.

159

mean that I endorse their use. This list is given as a comparison only and should be studied for what it is worth. Please understand that I am not endorsing Berg's theories."[33] Thus, the table was never meant to be some kind of mucusless versus mucus-forming foods chart, as some mistakenly believe. The chapter is more of an attempt to illustrate his alkaline versus acid-forming food theories using the work of his peers, although many of the items that are identified as acid-binding are not at all. The only foods that are truly acid-binding are fruits and green, leafy vegetables.

Nuts, in case you were confused, are mucus-forming. Confusion arises from a discrepancy in the book. In Lesson XI of the *Mucusless Diet,* it said that "all fruits, raw or cooked, also nuts and green-leaf vegetables, are mucus-free." Then, in Lesson XXI it says, "All nuts are too rich in protein and fat and should be eaten only in winter, and then only sparingly. Nuts should be chewed together with some dried sweet fruits or honey, never with juicy fruits, because water and fat do not mix." There are a couple possible explanations for the discrepancy. First, when compared with meat and dairy, nuts are *relatively* mucusless. For people coming from a meat-eating reality, nuts are a profound improvement. Another explanation is that the editor, Fred Hirsch, added nuts to the list of mucusless foods in the abovementioned statement. Hirsch takes certain editorial liberties throughout the book, and will even refer to Ehret in some instances.

In regard to the pepper and any condiments, if you crave it, eat it; but if you do not, do not. Again, do not sweat the small stuff. The way I look at it is that if I am filthy enough to digest it and I crave it, then I'll still eat it (within reason). This has served me well because it is impossible for me to eat foods that I used to eat. There will be no falling back as far as meat because it would probably kill me, or at least make me dreadfully ill. Plus, I know that whenever I do eat any mucus, I will be completely wasted, unable to function or think straight (high).

And for Little Joey: Keep the faith. Know that you are the vanguard and that eventually your peers will have to travel down the path you are traveling. The most important thing for you to do is to practice the diet. You do not have to explain or prove yourself to anybody. When I started the diet at school, it was hard because all of a sudden I had no way of relating to anybody. Before the diet, I had been the life of the

---

33. Ehret, *MDHS* 1994.

party, and as I came down from mucus I did miss this. None of my friends understood why I was doing what I was doing, and I learned quickly not to waste my time explaining. I'm not saying don't talk about the diet, but you don't have to offer information if you don't want to. After a while, when someone would ask me about the diet, I would just kind of brush it off acting like it was just another diet. Now, as these YOUNG people come to me sick with questions, they have to pay for a consultation, which I find to be important because people tend to not value information without paying for it. So stay strong and commune with your other friend who practices the diet. Eventually you will be brought together with others who also want to pursue superior health.

Peace, Love, and Breath!

-Professor Spira

Getting off Tobacco

Sent by Tim Wader on Monday, January 2, 2006 9:27 AM

Hi Spira!

Well, hopefully, today will be my last day of tobacco use. I was just wondering, what method or approach did you personally use to eliminate this awful burden from your life? How did you do it?

God Bless

Tim

Sent by Professor Spira on Monday, January 2, 2006 9:27 AM

Greetings Tim!

To eliminate tobacco and alcohol, I basically had faith in the system. I did not try to force myself to quit. I understood that as long as those poisons were in my bloodstream, I would crave them. My focus was on changing my physiology to the point where I would get severely sick from the use of intoxicants. Plus, I transitioned gently and comfortably. The longer I transitioned with the diet, the less I craved the intoxicants. Instead of a pack a day, I did a pack a week. Then I stopped cigarettes and used "freaked" Black and Mild's exclusively (a "freaked" Black and Mild is one with the carbon paper taken out of it)—first, once a day; then once a week, a month, etc. Finally, the fateful day came when I had a psychological flaw that enabled me to reach for a mild that made me feel so sick I knew that my body was done with the drug. I had a similar experience with alcohol. The key is to put everything into the slow and permanent change of your physiology. Instead of putting my willpower into ignoring my tobacco cravings, I put my discipline into lemon enemas and fruit. For me, this proved to be effective.

Peace, Love, and Breath!

-Spira

Sent by Tim Wader on Monday, January 2, 2006 9:27 AM

Hi Spira!

Interesting. I was kind of thinking along the same lines, actually, because I remembered Arnold's comments as well, matching yours on

162

how the diet will eventually cause your body to reject what is bad for it. That sounds like a much more secure, smooth/comfortable/non-stress to the body, and a permanent approach, really. I have never heard of Freaked Black and Mild's. Does the user take the carbon paper out, or are they actually purchased that way under a special brand/type name?

God Bless

-Tim

Sent by Professor Spira on Monday, January 2, 2006 9:27 AM

Tim,

The user takes the carbon paper out. It is actually a difficult task unless you know how to do it. I was very good at doing it and could do it in a matter of minutes. It is a popular stimulant in the young party scene that I was very much a part of. I would not recommend them to anyone, especially if they have never smoked them. I used it in my transition since I liked them more than cigarettes, but I have seen others get into them and get stuck. Of course, I recommend moving away from tobacco as fast as possible. The point is to acknowledge the addiction but not beat up yourself. The power of your intention to quit, coupled with the mucusless diet, is incredibly potent.

Peace, Love, and Breath!

-Spira

Sent by the Wader Family on Tuesday, January 3, 2006 3:56 AM

Oh, good thing you told me that part. Maybe it's best I did stay away from that part. I would agree to let the diet handle this issue for me. It has already happened with several other food items that I used to love to eat! I can no longer even stand to be in the same room now, as the scent just makes me ill. I would imagine, as the tissues in my body are cleansed deeper, the same will happen with the tobacco and coffee. We did find a "claimed" China non-acidic, organic, Free Trade coffee with only 9 percent or less caffeine level in it. It claims the pH levels to be 7.3 to 7.5. This may help with transitioning off that eventually, too. Like you said, keep it simple, don't sweat/stress the small stuff (even though this stuff, especially tobacco, is probably not really considered small); the power of the body and the diet will work it out in time. You are such a pleasure to talk with Spira, thank you for being there.

I hope your New Year is starting out magnificently and the power of the diet and God be with you.

Please, keep us up to date and posted on any news.

God Bless

-Tim, Samantha, and Little Joey

Questions about Water and Fasting

Friday, January 6, 2006 6:02 AM

Hi Spira!

Today, my stomach was having terrible discomfort after the lemona, along with a lot of fermentation going on after that, and I was telling Samantha basically the same thing. I told her that the lemons must have reached another layer of built-up waste in my intestines that it really, really doesn't like. In fact, it's 2:30 a.m. right now and I can still feel the lemon juice very much at work, as it should be ;-).

I can definitely understand that long fasts and long fruit/raw dieting right now would not be very efficient, because there needs to be actual elimination and not just excretion/shrinking from the fasts. I am still fasting, along with Samantha and Ant, though, but we have extended the period between each one. We were fasting about every fourth day prior to your post suggesting to slow down the transition, but now we'll fast after about every full week to 2 weeks, which will bring the fast to only about twice a month to give our intestines a break. I'm fasting about 3 days each time. Is it true that a fast doesn't really become fully efficient/effective until after the third day? When you said that fasting "then becomes" a result of an unobstructed body, do you mean that once the body is cleansed, fasting then becomes basically automatic, as eating becomes less necessary and easier to handle?

I forgot to mention that I also weighed myself today, and after being pretty steady for a while at around 154/156 pounds (dropping pretty quick from the 190 or so I started at), I weighed in at just under 150 lbs now. Samantha seemed a bit worried, but I'm not too much. I was always around 148 or so with a 30/31-inch waist when I was young. I'm now a very loose 34, very loose indeed ;-). I told her that I believe the diet/cleansing is beginning to move deeper into the tissues of my body, removing the mucus/pus obstructions by moving on to the daily fruit/fruit salad lunches and vegetable salads with baked or steamed vegetable dinners, along with a periodic slice of wheat toast with almond/peanut butter or a very-well-baked potato seasoned with sesame/almond butter. Tie together with that the daily lemon enemas. Don't know where the weight will steady at this time, but would it be safe to assume this is what's happening (deeper tissue cleansing, thus the added weight loss?)

Have a perfect day and God Bless!

Sincerely,

-Tim, Samantha, and Little Joey

Email sent by Spira on Sunday, January 8, 2006 7:27 AM

Tim,

You wrote:

> Is it true that a fast doesn't really become fully efficient/effective until after the third day? When you said below that fasting "then becomes" a result of an unobstructed body, do you mean that once the body is cleansed, fasting then becomes basically automatic, as eating becomes less necessary and easier to handle?

Actually, we look at the entire *Mucusless Diet Healing System* as one long fast. As Ehret says, anytime that you decrease the amount of food intake into the body it is essentially fasting. Throughout the entire diet, you are slowly eliminating foods and quantities, therefore refining one's diet into a permanent fast. Of course, in conversation, we use the word to identify periods when we abstain from solid food, but a big-picture analysis will be of assistance to your inquiry about the days. The length of a fast is not as important as the way in which you break it. A 1-day fast broken with fruit or a salad is much better than a 7-day fast broken with corn chips and beans. Many fasters try to fast for long periods of time only to uncontrollably binge, therefore ruining the fast. Strive to break the fast correctly. Setting up good habits now will be very beneficial for the future. The cleaner the body gets, fasting will become the rule and not the exception.

In regard to your question about water, distilled water is the cleanest water available for us to use. Remember, we do not believe that the body is absorbing and assimilating any minerals from water. It is merely a tool to be used to help "ring out" our dirty rags—called tissues. As you research waters, you will find that waters other than distilled go through some questionable procedures. Brother Air speaks of a documentary he watched on water that shows how ash gets into many bottled spring waters. At the end of the day, the medical establishment wants you to believe in erroneous theories so that you will buy steroid-pumped toilet

166

water. The human body is not made of 90 percent water. Try to cut your arm and drain some water into a cup. While you are at it, get some vitamins out too. Brother Air did not drink any water during his 8½-month fast. I'm not saying not to drink water, just understand that the perception of its necessity, like food's, is erroneous. As Brother Air says, this thing is all about the bloodstream and its plight to become clean.

Hopefully, everything is going well with you. I will talk to you soon.

Health Is Wealth!

-Professor Spira

Email sent by Tim Wader on Sunday, January 8, 2006 7:27 AM

Hi Spira!

Wow, those were some interesting answers, especially your reply on water. Very different from what is out there today, that's for sure!

Your fasting reply makes great sense. I'll have to keep focused on the long-term functionality of the diet. It makes absolute sense that "how" one breaks the fast would be more important, because if that is done improperly, like you mentioned, the fast would have been for nothing and could even become dangerous. We usually follow the chopped cabbage, chopped celery, and prune dish. Then, if nothing happens after about an hour, some prune juice. That usually does the job; but if not, either way, an enema (now lemon enemas) is done.

That was very interesting about the water. I loved your example of trying to cut off your arm and fill a cup of water! No kidding, if we were 90 percent water, one would have to believe that there would be more water than blood coming from the wound. Interesting! It makes sense, though, because even when they tell you to drink the "required" amount of water each day, they also tell you that drinking too much water is also not good—much like food intake, as you already mentioned. I am sure that the "profits of the water industry" have played some influence, much like the dairy and cattlemen's associations played in promoting proteins/meat/eggs/milk/food charts, etc. Wow! One has to energize, jump for joy, and become zealous in learning the truth!

Everything is going well here. I will be breaking my 3-day fast today. Samantha and Little Joey are doing very well also. Our daughter, Jane, is also (without really knowing it, but we're noticing a difference) eating more toward the diet with more vegetables/fruits/juices, along with some of her normal poor diet, thus actually in a (hidden from herself) slow, progressive transition.

Have an amazing, successful day!

God Bless

-Tim

Pain from Poor Food Combinations and Lemon Enemas

Sent by Tim Wader on Wednesday, January 18, 2006 8:32 AM

Hi Spira!

We hope that everything has been going very well back there!

I just wanted to stop in to check in with you on how we've been doing. First, I think you'll be happy to hear that I have built up to 12 lemons per day for the lemon enemas so far! :) Other than the normal fermentation/gastric issues from the bacteria in the intestines, is it normal to have intense/pretty much painful gastric build up? Sometimes painful to even walk normally...it kind of stops you in your tracks, the pain. Is this from the lemon enemas for some reason? We have been trying different food combination techniques to try to keep it under control/normal, but it seems to be only working on some days. I usually wake up at around 2 p.m. each day (due to schedule), take my enema at around 5-6 p.m. Shortly after, about 30 minutes or so, I have my fruit salad. If still hungry, I'll have toasted wheat bread with or without almond/peanut butter about 30 minutes after. Then I'll eat a salad with a different dressing each day, at around 3 a.m., followed by a steamed vegetable. The gastric problems seem to appear about an hour or so before lunch or not too long thereafter and last until around 5-6 a.m. Samantha has been complaining about an intense amount of gastric build up too, as well as Little Joey. Is this normal? From the lemon enemas or some other reason? Is there any way to tame it back to a normal level, not so intense/painful? Will it eventually calm itself down back to normal on its own? Is there really anything to the food-combining information that is out there?

Samantha and Little Joey are moving along really well, keeping steady! Samantha is having about 2 to 3 days of low to no body pain, with about 1-2 days of really bad pain in between. It used to be a daily problem, so she's very hopeful in seeing some progress! :) Little Joey is doing well, except some pretty intense skin breakouts, especially in the webs of his fingers and acne on his face. Little Joey is currently at the fourth 2-week menu schedule from the book that he is choosing to go by. Sam is somewhat in the third 2-week menu zone. ;)

Well, other than that, I thought you might like to hear how we were doing/progressing...steady and still very committed! :) Besides being pressed by work times and short play times, we're all doing well.

169

We hope everyone back there is doing very well and things are progressively and successfully moving along!

Talk with you soon.

God Bless!

Sincerely,

-Tim, Samantha, and Little Joey

Friday, January 20, 2006 3:51 AM

Hi Spira!

Well, we believe we figured out the cause of the gastric problem. The day I wrote you, it was the worst for me, and we determined that it must have been the bowl of cherries I had for lunch. The day prior and the next 2 days after, in following food-combining principles, there has only been the normal, minimum of gastric issue generated. Also, in researching further with Samantha and Ant, they have not been following any food-combining principles, mixing acidic with alkaline, etc., thus causing enzymatic problems in their intestines. They said they are going to work to improve that.

Just wanted to update you on what we have figured out so far.

Have a perfect, healthy day!

God Bless

-Tim, Samantha, and Little Joey

Sunday, January 22, 2006 12:07 PM

Greetings,

Nice to hear from you all. Sorry it took so long to get back. I've been focusing on the fast that I started last week. There are about five of us fasting all at the same time (and the weatherman wonders why we are having unseasonably warm temperatures ;-). You did a nice job with analyzing your gas problems. During any kind of elimination, no matter how small or big, it is of the utmost importance to stop and think about it. You know that you only have about three different courses of action: be more aggressive, less aggressive, or stop eating all together. Fruits are

170

extremely aggressive and when mixed with the toxic waste in the body create a great deal of gas. Really aggressive lemon enemas can create the same results. However, sometimes it may be prudent to pursue a more aggressive elimination, whenever you can handle it. To make the elimination less aggressive, use less lemons in your enemas (and sometimes just do plain distilled water enemas).

Furthermore, it is very important that you be mindful of the order in which you eat things and the mixtures. Let as much time pass as possible between fruit meals and vegetable meals, unless you are eating a fruit-and-vegetable meal as described by Ehret. Try not to drink until well after your meal. Do not overcook your vegetables. Overcooked vegetables are starchy and will find ways to make you feel very uncomfortable. I would also try to eat the toast during your vegetable meal, far away from the fruit. The toast really needs to be eaten with vegetables to be eliminated properly. Eating toast and nut butter after fruit will not leave a happy stomach.

With all this said, it is to be expected to have some gas problems. Some people's physiological eliminations occur through gas, while others go through intense physical pain. The key psychological factor you must keep reminding yourself about is that, in our current pathological condition, it is normal to be a bit uncomfortable and sometimes in pain as we eliminate. We must pay reparations for the pain that we did not experience immediately after eating wrong foods in the past. Luckily, a solid understanding of the systematic nature of the diet, coupled with experience, will give you the tools you need to go through your eliminations with as much ease as is possible.

Peace, Love, and Breath!

-Professor Spira

Sunday, January 22, 2006 12:07 PM

Hi Spira!

That is awesome to have a team fast going on! That generates a lot of support around you.

We have been doing as you said to me the very first time, "Listen to your professors and study long." We are indeed committed! When this problem began to really progress, it brought us into the study of food combining. In any of our studies outside of Arnold's writings, we always work to remain mindful of remaining focused on his teachings and not steering off into another direction, thus defeating our diet.

From our studies, we did make several adjustments. We did move the eating of our toast to the vegetable meal, about 20 to 30 minutes post-meal. We've focused on whether the breads are whole or sprouted; if we're eating the sprouted, then it's eaten plain (without the nut butter) to ensure that mildly starchy does not mix with the proteins. If we have a well-baked potato instead of toast, then it's eaten with a non-starchy, green-leaf vegetable topping instead of any kind of nut butter, etc. Our mixtures of fruits for our fruit salads are carefully selected to ensure the best enzymatic reaction/flow within the GI tract. We've also learned not to grate/shred up our salads as much. We've also become very mindful of the dressing uses/mixtures as well. I'm sure doing this is also helping further in the broom action. We're also waiting longer times after meals to drink any fluids. We're focusing more on the best steaming/cooking times for the foods as well to ensure they're not quickly switching over to the starchy/toxic side. The times have been cut back significantly actually. These methods are truly helping!

Samantha actually discovered something new going on with me just yesterday. I had the front of my shirt pulled up to take care of a persistent itchy feeling in the lower rib area on both sides. She noticed many bright red, some not so bright a red, speckles/freckles spread all over those areas (skin surface over the liver, upper GI and over to the pancreas/spleen area) that had not been near that prominent before. I did have a few in this area and the stomach area in the past, but not near as large/bold or prominent. So, we've been researching since last night trying to figure that out.

We definitely agree (and I keep reminding Samantha, Little Joey, and myself at times actually) that we do have to pay for our sins of prior poor eating/lifestyle habits. The positive thing is, we indeed know that the direction we're taking is the only direction to take and that whatever we experience physiologically, etc., along the way to reach the goal of paradisiac health is absolutely worth it!

Well, I best get going here. I'll be starting a fast myself tonight when I return back to work. I'll be trying for another 3- to 5-day fast.

It was an absolute pleasure, as it always is, to hear from you Spira, and it's a comfort to know that you are in fact OK. Talk with you soon.

Have a wonderful, healthy and very successful day!

God Bless,

-Tim, Samantha, and Little Joey

Doing Daily Enemas and Questions about the 80/10/10 Diet

Sent by Tim Wader on Monday, January 30, 2006 2:42 AM

Hi Spira!

Hope all is going well with everyone back there!

We were wondering if you, or any of the other professors, have heard of, looked into or know anything of the 80/10/10 Diet out there? When looking into proper food combining, we ended up running into this diet, which appears a lot like ours except they appear to be eating a lot of fruits and veggies, less seeds and nuts, trying to get to a 80 percent carb, 10 percent protein, 10 percent fat (of the total daily calorie need for each one's particular metabolism) per day, intake. It appears though, that they are eating immense amounts of fruits and greens to get there (meeting their daily calorie requirement). We just wanted to know what, if any, experiences or knowledge you all had of it back there.

Also, what are your opinions on taking enemas every day? Is this something that will have to be done basically forever or is there an ending point to them eventually? We've been getting information about how the intestine can basically become inflamed, swollen, create bacteria imbalances and possibly the muscles that move the waste toward elimination can weaken or forget how to function properly. What are the thoughts on this information back there?

Also, I started feeling dehydrated and wondered if it was the lemon enemas. I've decreased the amount of lemons I use, to find out.

Must go for now. Please tell everyone we said Hi and to take care!

God Bless,

-Tim

Email sent by Spira on Tuesday, February 7, 2006 5:40 AM

Greetings!

Things over here have been going great. Brother Air has been fasting for the past 4 months, and I for almost 3 weeks. It feels great to be not eating again!

In response to your question about the 80/10/10 Diet, we have found many of these kinds of diets problematic because most do not deal with how the body truly operates. I do not believe in the calorie theory, which is a primary focus on the 80/10/10. With that said, as a raw-fruit-centric diet, it is more advanced than many. But, in all of the literature I have come across, I have yet to find anybody talk about the human body being an air-gas engine. Even people who claim to be breathaireans talk about being fed by something other than air, for example Prahlad Jani (Indian fakir and faster) claims that he is fed nectar through the palette in his mouth by an angel (I cannot help but wonder if this nectar is really mucus from his tissue system). Nobody is acknowledging that the body is an air-gas engine and providing a systematic method to eliminate the waste that we have accumulated through generations of wrong eating. Although the diet may be looked at as a particular level on the transition, the "how" and "why" of eating is very problematic. Within such dietetic paradigms, people eat for calories and nutrition. In Ehret's paradigm, one eats primarily for the purpose of elimination, and calorie and protein theories are unnecessary and potentially harmful. I'm open to exploring new information, but it has to at least be in line with, or go beyond, the information that Ehret has provided. To this date, I have not found anything that goes further than Ehret. However, it is not surprising that nobody has been able to really deal with the air-gas engine fact because this must be experienced to truly be understood. The art of the transition must be practiced on an exceptionally high level to experience such elevated stages.

The fact that the body exists solely on air did not completely click with me until I became clean enough to do some longer fasts. Unfortunately, the amount of time that it takes to get clean enough to experience the body at peace with no other stimulants varies from person to person. No matter how physiologically advanced somebody is, it is all about transition. This diet is the art form of all art forms. The patient's determination and mindset is important to practicing this diet. One must try to stay as focused as possible because it is easy to get sidetracked. Please remember that certain members of our community, like Brother Air, have proven beyond a reasonable doubt that the nutrition theory, vitamin theory, protein theory, and any other theories about the health and well-being of the human body established by the medical "witch" science are totally wrong. On our own bodies, we have proven that it is indeed an air-gas engine and that the only way to return back to this state is to retrace our steps through transitioning from whence we came. Understand that the use of food loosens and eliminates dead matter from the body, enabling the bloodstream to more

175

effectively use oxygen. As the bloodstream is oxygenated, it is truly cleaned—so in essence, food only helps get rid of waste that prevents the bloodstream from cleansing itself. Once the bloodstream is clean enough, air alone will be the only stimulant that you need.

In terms of food combinations, you must transition toward clear combinations as specified in the *Mucusless Diet*. You must clearly define your goals and use recommendations from the book and your own experience to transition toward them. My goal is to achieve freedom from wrong eating. In order to do this, I must first become totally mucusless, then a fruit eater, and finally an air-eater. These stages are physiological and will just happen naturally when the mechanics of the *Mucusless Diet Healing System* are adhered to. Remember to not be hard on yourself. Our ancestors have been killing themselves with mucus for thousands of generations. We must be patient as we embark on a journey 180 degrees in the opposite direction.

In regards to your mentioning your feeling weak sometimes, I applaud your efforts. This means that you are eliminating waste. Remember that Ehret explained that most people who start the diet at first feel wonderful and then come down and stay down a while. Our challenge is negotiating our newly unstimulated state with the 9-to-5 mucus world. Some days you just need to be able to lie down and eliminate. Your peers do not understand that before something can strengthen, it will weaken; and the diet demands the utmost focus, time, and energy. For us, the diet is the top priority. Our jobs and activities all revolve around the diet. We are not rich, but we always have exactly what we need. In fact, last year Brother Air's wife went through a 2-month long elimination where she had to quit her job and just focus on her elimination. Brother Air picked up the slack and kept everything together. There are similar stories within the community. The important thing is to understand that there is nothing more important than your health and that it should not ever be placed second. My experiences have proven to me that when I honestly put my all into the diet, everything I need comes to me. The diet will challenge your perception of what you "want" and "need." I want all kinds of things, but I know that I must strive to want what I need. When I need energy to go make money or write a 10-page paper, I have it. Before I submitted to the diet 100 percent, it was very hard for me to negotiate in this world powered by mucus. It was as if the universe gave me an ultimatum to either pursue my health to its highest potential or to stay in mucus world. As soon as I wholeheartedly dedicated myself to pursuing superior health with the Muscusless Diet Healing System, all of the worldly struggles I was going through faded away. Bills were paid on time and my grades became flawless.

About the enemas: It is necessary to do enemas as long as our tissue systems are filled with pus and mucus. You can gain an understanding of how important enemas are by using the simple logic of cause and effect. Because I and my ancestors did something totally unnatural (putting solid matter into my human air-gas engine), I must do something equally unnatural on the opposite end until I can return to my perfect state. Everybody is sentenced to a different amount of time due to their personal mucus condition. It may take one person 30 years of enemas, it may take another 300. At this point, the time it takes is irrelevant; every human's current mucus condition demands a total lifestyle of transitioning with enemas. In regards to what critics say about enemas, how do they know? How did they become authorities on the subject when they haven't done enemas regularly for 30 years themselves? The symptoms they speak of come from about of a week of enemas with a patient who is not fasting or transitioning. They may also be using the chemical fleet enemas, which really irritate colons. An enema is incapable of creating bacteria and it is incapable of dehydrating you. Similarly, the mucus that you may spit out after eating an orange is not from the orange. All of these symptoms derive from foreign matter that has been in your bloodstream for thousands of years. When I started the diet, my mouth used to get so dry that it seemed absurd. Then I realized how salty my mucus is, and that my body is now in a serious eliminatory mode. To stay comfortable, I just drank as much juice as I needed. In regard to your discomfort, I believe that you did the perfect thing by lightening up on the lemons. Learning how to control and be less aggressive with your eliminations is an essential aspect of this art form. Consistency is the most important thing.

That's all for now. We encourage you and your family to keep on fighting the good fight. Understand that in time you will gain superior knowledge about the human body. You will be able to look no further than your own body when confronted with the many thousands of erroneous concepts and theories about how it works. But to experience the many joyous revelations your body has to offer you, it is important to stay focused on your goal of superior health.

Health is Wealth!

Professor Spira

Tuesday, February 7, 2006 5:40 AM

Hi Spira!

Congratulations on the fastings! Beautiful! We are both proud and happy for you both!

Thank you so much for such a wonderful post! It was most definitely encouraging and inspiring! We in fact did get into a regroup mode here. I read through the *Mucusless Diet Healing System* book again, slower, marking as I went. I then went back, making my highlights into an outline on our computer. I also printed it up and placed it in a three-ring binder. We now have a quick reference source to the book in two places. I am now reading *Rational Fasting* again and doing the same thing, which I will add the notes to the Fasting Lessons of the *MDHS* book outline. We are most definitely committed!

Samantha is still struggling with fatigue, weakness, hypoglycemic symptoms, female issues increased, but most definitely committed. Since the regroup, I pulled back a little, using more of the provided menus of the book for transition, trying to slow down the elimination some to help make it through the 9-5 as you mentioned. A little more challenging for me, as we have two children to care for and Samantha is out of working condition. So here, the 9-5 part is critical for me. The enemas indeed help. So, I was glad to read your positive, sensible response on that! I don't have an appendix, which I believe causes me some breakdown/bowel movement issues, therefore generating the abnormal means/need of assistance. We truly believe the human being is fully capable of living on air as food when its condition is right. There is no reasonable explanation why it would not! You are correct in your findings, that no other group out there goes as deep or as far as Arnold has! Like Arnold said, if it's not easily understood, then it's not the truth!

Thank you again, Spira, for the wonderful, wonderful post! You have NO idea how encouraging it was! Thank you! We are the only ones over here around us on the diet, so your encouragements with the incredible posts and readings of other Ehretists on the site who have been on the diet for some time is so very deeply helpful and from the heart appreciated with much gratefulness!

A word of encouragement from here…our daughter, Janet, has read the book all the way through on her own and now wants to restart the healing system with us! She now has a greater understanding of what we're working to do and why! :)))

178

Please pass on our greetings and congrats to Brother Air and the rest of the community! Whenever we hear from you, we indeed feel the energy of all of you all the way over here! It's incredible!

God Bless all of you!

Sincerely,

-Tim, Samantha, and Little Joey

The Waders Learning to Navigate the Transition

Tuesday, February 7, 2006 7:04 AM

Hi Spira!

I thought I should add a couple of notes to my previous post, maybe to help better explain at least my situation. In addition to what I wrote:

> I was eating only raw fruit salads for lunch with a raw salad (minimal to no dressings/herbs/spices on it), starches gone, and even began to cut out the cooked vegetable portion of the meal. Way too much, way too quick! Thank goodness I caught myself, as I was feeling absolutely miserable and almost unable to function at all. I've regrouped and am feeling better, eating only once per day and will work back into fasting 2 days, eat 3 or 4; then 3 days, eat 3 or 4, and so on.

I believe what was happening is that I was actually developing a fear of putting even more mucus/toxins with these foods into my system/body than I was eliminating, developing a fear of not succeeding long term. So, I basically psychologically scared myself away from all those parts of the transition foods, necessary for a proper, slowly regulated transition. Is that kind of what you see here?

Also, one additional issue that Samantha has been uncomfortable with is when she fasts and does the enemas, she seems to have endless "trots," liquidy bowel movements. She has been having these a lot throughout the day since on the diet, as well as a really bad pain in the chest/heart, especially when fasting. In the past, she took an incredible amount of vitamins, herbal pills/potions for her conditions. She also drank an incredible amount of goat milk each day, along with goat protein, homemade goat yogurts, and acidophilus in a yogurt form. She then ate many times throughout the day due to her hypoglycemia, eating snack foods (i.e., chips, crackers, cookies, basically a lot of junk food) to keep going. Don't know if all this has to do with her having trouble, but I do remember Arnold mentioning that one will experience many sensations including heart palpitations during a fast. When she feels these, would it be wise to break the fast at that point, try an enema first? She has had so many health issues for so, so very long; trying so diligently toward feeling better health. She deserves to make it through this system to feel a true superior health! I just want to be careful and also ensure that the system is properly implemented to ensure a superior health success.

Have an incredibly healthy, successful and wonderful day!

God Bless!

Sincerely,

-Tim

Email Sent by Prof. Spira on Monday, February 13, 2006 8:10 PM

Greetings Wader Family!

I am pleased to hear that Janet has read the book again and is pursuing the diet. She will be much envied by future generations who will wish that they had the opportunity to begin the diet at such a young age. I always tell a person that no matter what their age is, the time to start pursuing the *Mucusless Diet* is now, because it will not be any easier later.

In regard to your concerns about the transition, it sounds like you are all on the right track. One thing that Brother Air always says to people is that you could be on the transition diet for 30 or 40 years, but you will still be here. At this point, it is not necessary to try to rush certain transitional foods away for good, but focus on the mechanical operations of the body during the transition. You will find that over time, the transitional mucuses become irritating, and you will no long be able to eat them with any comfort. But with this said, strive to eat only what you feel you truly need. Keep on taking baby steps. If you are eating two pieces of toast with your meal, try to eat just one and a half. If you are accustomed to nut butter, see what happens if you use a bit of raw dressing or tomato sauce. These kinds of small transitions are really what make the transition an artistic science. The more you can listen to your body and what it needs, the more effective your decisions will become.

In regard to Samantha, she needs to really try to pursue transitional foods that make it comfortable for her over the long haul. Some people are able to grind their teeth through a fast and come out on the other end with a great deal of her type of symptoms gone. The best thing to do is to stay on the transition for a long time. The heart pain during fasting is probably from pus and chemicals recirculating in the body,

181

especially from pharmaceuticals. I would recommend vegetable meals of steamed broccoli, salads with romaine lettuce, and a piece of wheat toast when desired to slow down the elimination. One of the approaches that I have been very successful with is finding meal combinations that work and sticking to them for long lengths of time. When I saw how effective steamed broccoli, collard greens, and salads were, I would not deviate from this form of vegetable meal until my body moved me on to something else. Such a regimen would often lead to an all-fruit fast.

I did 3 months straight with steamed broccoli and salads being my only vegetable meals. I know how attached we are to eating varieties of foods, but varieties do not eliminate as well as sticking to very simple combinations that have proven to eliminate well in your own body. Some of the diarrhea will have to be tolerated for awhile, but the proper vegetables can help sweep some stuff out more effectively. One thing that may be causing the diarrhea is the fallout of the enema assaults. As you get a few months into the enemas, you begin to break down new layers of filth in the intestines. What happens is the filth on the walls of the intestines absorbs the liquid from the enema. You may put a whole bag in but feel like nothing is coming back out. As it gets absorbed, the filth starts to loosen up, creating watery discharges. Personally, I found steamed broccoli and big salads help sweep the absorbed debris more comfortably. You see, the broccoli is important because raw lettuce alone may not be heavy enough to effectively sweep encumbered intestinal walls.

Peace, Love, and Breath!

-Prof. Spira

182

Questions about the Master Cleanse Method

Email sent by Prof. Spira on Monday, February 13, 2006 8:10 PM

Hi Spira!

I definitely appreciated your comments on the transition phase. We have definitely regrouped here, and are focusing closely on our transition, taking it slowly. We diverted and converted too quickly, and our bodies let us know that very well! Our focus will be, as you mentioned, to learn to eat less first, as we go along, prior to moving on to progressively eliminating particular foods. We have been working hard in recognizing which foods are irritating and eliminating those. Samantha has been working diligently on lessening the "variety" effect, but where we live, good foods are seemingly difficult to find; and when they are, they tend to be significantly higher priced. So, before things go bad, there's a tendency to varietize the salads more, especially. We are working on that ;). Ant is in love with his nut-butter toast though, that's for sure ;)! A growing, teenage boy :)!

Janet hasn't quite kick-started on the diet yet. She has read the book fully and now understands the principles. We're not trying to push her, as she would have more success initiating it on her own, but we are hopeful. She wants to finish the foods she has available here for her already and then initiate. We told her that if she likes, we could still begin to transition her along with those foods in the meantime, so it wouldn't feel like such an impact to her. We've been kind of doing it for her really, unbeknownst to her ;-).

In my prior post to you, I brought up a cleansing fast which we read about on the Arnold Ehret site that other Ehretists on there have done and are doing. It is called the Master Cleanse [MC], otherwise known as the Lemonade diet. Have you or anyone in the community heard of it and is it a fasting cleanse that would be recommended to perform? In my research on it, it has had tremendous success for those who smoke and drink coffee, etc., which was my personal drive for wanting to give it a try, as many have said going through it, by the time it's complete, the desires/cravings for those things completely disappear midstream! If yourself or anyone in the community are aware of it and believe it would be an OK fast to undergo, please let us know, and as soon as I have completed reading through the supplementary book on it, we will give it a try!

Spira, it is always SO wonderful hearing from you and please know that it is always very deeply appreciated and that we are incredibly proud of you and the community there in all you've accomplished and are pursuing! To be a working part of it all, must be and would be, a blessing indeed! We have no doubts in the future successes of the efforts taking place! You are all in our prayers and may all of the winds of the negative, powerful worldly influences which have caused mankind such great hindrance, look upon all the efforts going on there in awe and have absolutely no strength within it to even impose one breath against its work!

God Bless our dear friend!

-Tim, Samantha, Little Joey, and Janet

Thursday, February 23, 2006 4:00 PM

Greetings Wader Family!

In regard to your question about the Master Cleanse, nobody in our camp has ever used that explicit method. Others have asked us about it and we feel that in many cases it is used as an attempt to try to take a shortcut. Its methods, as is every other diet to my knowledge, are in some way encapsulated by the *Mucusless Diet Healing System*. I can roll with the lemon and lime juice, but in my opinion the use of such stimulants as maple syrup, tea, and cayenne pepper will only stir up and irritate the mucus in the system. If you are going to fast, I would recommend sticking to Ehret's methods. I do know of one person who got into the Master Cleanser after giving up on Ehret's writings (he never actually tried it). It seemed that he enjoyed some short-term success, but now he eats worse than he did before and uses an inhaler to deal with the mucus in his lungs. If you ask me, doing a long but permanent transition is much more effective than any attempt at speeding up the transition. Striving for one's full potential within the confines of the *Mucusless Diet* is very different than attempting some kind of shortcut. As Ehret said, *nature's mills grind slowly*, but they definitely grind. In my opinion, the methods of the Master Cleanser are flawed. However, if somebody was trying to do it, I would not deter them, especially if they are just starting to become conscious about their health. I would recommend that they read the *Mucusless Diet* first before engaging in eating syrup and cayenne pepper, but I would leave it at that. Eating fruit that will transform into syrup (waste) in the body seems

184

more rational than eating the waste material formed from fruit. Furthermore, it is okay to enjoy the transition; I enjoy eating fruit, but syrup, cayenne pepper, and water sounds pretty nasty to me. As Ehret says, anything that is not simple and rational is humbug. Brother Air has watched people attempt to practice the diet for the past 30 years and has observed that most people who try to incorporate methods of other diets usually fail to sustain any long-term results. I understand that it can be confusing since there are so many different diets, theories, and points of view out there; but it has always been my personal philosophy to get into one thing and focus on it long enough to see if it does what it says it is supposed to do. For right now, I have tunnel vision for Ehret's work. If somebody can turn me on to a system and philosophy that is more profound than Ehret's, my interest may be perked; but until then, I intend to find out about $V = P - O$ and learn more about the nature of my air-gas engine.

I hope that everything is going well with you and your family. I will talk to you soon.

Peace, Love, and Breath be unto you all!

-Professor Spira

Thursday, February 23, 2006 4:00 PM

Hi Spira!

Whew, that was close really ;). I was planning on March 1 to try this! I was definitely thinking along the lines you described, but also read how others/Ehretists had done it. I still had reservations, much like the ones you described, but I have been having such a difficult time in giving up the tobacco habit, which I feel has got to be having negative effects on my progress. I read some very positive notes on how the MC worked very well for those hooked on tobacco and coffee especially and had a deep desire to want to give it a try to rid myself of these awful burdens. I still wasn't sure though because of the rapid detox process and the comments made on knowing when the fast was complete: until the tongue is pink. I read that and a red flag went up, remembering Arnold's writings on his warnings of some who recommend fasting until the tongue is pink and the negatives of that! So, I was looking for the experience of other Ehretists to hopefully come to a conclusion/support of either going ahead with it or not. I will indeed adhere to your thoughts below.

We regard the knowledge and experience of you and your community there very highly! It is very much in line with my original pondering on the matter, along with Arnold's comments; we will stick to the program. I am hoping that the diet will eventually bring my body to the point of absolutely rejecting tobacco so terribly that I will not be able to tolerate it whatsoever. Much like other things it has already done that with.

Thank you SO much for confirming my thoughts on the Master Cleanse Spira! You are a blessing to our family indeed!

Peace and Superior Health to you and all in the community there our dear friend! Please tell everyone we said "Hi" and we pray for endless success for them all!

God Bless!

Sincerely,

-Tim

VOLUME THREE (Advanced Literature)

Chapter 6: Correspondence between Professor Spira and Cy

Greetings!

Email from Cy on May 5, 2008

Let me reiterate my pleasure in hearing from you. Funny you connected to me through an Arnold Ehret book. I randomly stumbled upon him at a health food store in Brooklyn called Perelandra. I had heard of his name, and the books were super cheap, so I picked up two and found that they reinforced and expanded on the raw-food concepts I was incorporating into my life.

Your music and media concepts sound delightful and wonderfully consciousness raising (diluting the lies); though I have yet to listen, I will. Further, I'll be in touch as I am developing an educational website centered around holistic and earth-foods nutrition with a focus on low cost and feasibility, and centered around people of color and people in exploited and postcolonial contexts. I would love to include your perspective.

Quisqueya—Not sure if you know, but I live currently in the Dominican Republic (what the indigenous of the isle called "Quisqueya"). I'm here for about another 11 months (creator permitting) on a bit of a personal journey whose trajectory I could have never predicted. Being healthy is culturally difficult but materially easy, as the land is rich and its products fresher and generally cheaper. Prior to this, I lived in New York where I was quite the foo-foo raw foodist, dining at my favorite raw restaurants whenever I felt the whim. Transition to island life has been interesting, to say the least.

Your personal rediscovery of your radiant, intended self is amazing! Living examples, that's what people like you are like, timeless individuals who live natural truth and telebeam it to others. I think my raw foodism and purist/earth substance way of life was inspired by my desire for more in my life, to transcend the disease states, which have burrowed their way into my family line (diabetes, heart disease, alcoholism) and those that have tried to pass themselves down to me (thyroid disorder, depression). I was vegan for 5 years before I adopted a raw-food lifestyle and way of thinking. I had a macrobiotic midpoint, which though not attuned to my system, helped me eliminate basically all non-earth foods from my diet; but then raw foods were the only thing to even begin helping me to deal with the surface of my struggle for thyroid balance.

I am glad to have connected with you. Your statement, "How can young musicians be expected to learn how to play jazz if the music is tucked away in temples of debauchery and diversion?" is the truth and could be panned out to a lot of other spheres of life. Keep the jazz coming, and I'll keep my ears clean for proper listening.

Much peace and positive energy to you,

-Cy

Email from Prof. Spira on May 11, 2008 at 5:55 am

Greetings Cy!

Reading *Autobiography of a Yogi* was a monumental turning point for me. I was a junior in high school and desperately searching for my purpose and the meaning of life. Although publically I was perceived to be a strong and popular football playin', Eagle Scout achieving, Louis Armstrong Award winning success story, I was not satisfied. This discontentment urged me to dive deeper into more abstract realities and music became my primary vehicle. I began to take private trombone lessons from Eddie Morgan, an ex-Vegas jazzman who had practiced Kriya Yoga for over 30 years. He mentioned Yogananda's (1971) book to me and I was very intrigued. The next week, I surprised him by having already read the book and sent away for the Fellowship's yoga literature. I was studying and experimenting with an amalgam of

188

existential activities and vegetarian concepts were finally on the table, thanks to Yogananda.

When it was time for college, I decided to pursue music, the ultimate consciousness raiser. I knew that I was not going to learn how to play African American music by only studying at a predominantly white institution, so I created my own curriculum that included field studies at black communal soundscapes: jazz clubs, after hour joints, churches, etc. I soon met the drummer Brother Air, who seemed to be one of the most authentic jazz musicians in the city. His passion for the music, coupled with his militant, no-nonsense attitude, is just what I was looking for in a black musical mentor. One day a few months after I had met Brother Air, we were sitting with some other musicians between sets at a club named Chez Nora in Covington, KY. He began to talk about health and how the body is the true instrument. He asserted that an artist's first priority, no matter what the art form, is the refinement of the real instrument, i.e., the human body. Then he started to talk about a fruit and vegetable diet and the elimination of pus and mucus from the body. His claim that the diet was the one and only cure for disease caught my interest. I really became curious when he told us that he had been eating nothing but fruit for the past year with much fasting.

We asked, "But what about protein and vitamins?" He quickly asserted that there is no more destructive myth known to man than the additive principle, or believing that the body needs foods to grow and operate properly. He explained that the only reason that we need to eat is to control our perpetual mucus elimination. Once our bodies are free of pus and mucus, it then becomes impossible to die of disease. Most people will agree that it is possible to go a day without food and water, but try to go 5 or 10 minutes without air. He expressed that the body is an AIR-GAS ENGINE, which, at the time, seemed like an abstract concept. It would take about a year of dedicated practicing of the *Mucusless Diet* to experience and understand my body as an air-gas engine; but the idea of a human being able to exist on nothing but fruit was very attractive and sensible to me.

While being a resident-advisor in a dorm, I began to practice the diet. This meant daily enemas in a public dorm bathroom stall and taking the fruit/vegetable "decorations" off of the lunch line to prepare and eat. I then thought about my yoga and meditation efforts and realized that I could never get anywhere because I always needed to blow my nose or spit out a mouthful of mucus. I soon realized that a

189

mucus-filled diet and body was holding me back from achieving my full physiological potential. Furthermore, I began to see how pathologically sick we humans really are from generations of pus- and mucus-poisoning ,and how it will take a very long time to undo this diabolical travesty. As I began to practice the diet, I dedicated myself to studying the experiences and techniques of its chief practitioners. Brother Air's entire family is formed around the *Mucusless Diet*, and I noted how much he and his family contributed to its practice.

How does one become mucusless? By adopting a rational, transitional lifestyle; and Brother Air's family are the exemplars of this. I quickly realized that I was privy to the interiority of one of the most important rediscoveries since gravity; that the body is an air-gas engine and we must engage in a rational, safe TRANSITION to our natural state. But, such a profound contribution has been made to the practice of the diet that I am of the opinion that it would be extremely hard to practice it without the unique insight of these pioneers. Despite the thousands of books sold, there are not too many people who can sustain the diet as a lifestyle.

In 2004, Brother Air began to do a long juice fast and I was able to bear witness to the feat. We were running around, playing music on the streets in Chicago, etc., and no one would have known that he had been fasting for the past 9 months if he hadn't told them. This was one of the most impactful experiences in my life. For the next 3 years, Brother Air would only eat for a total of 6 months. I would even get in on the action with three 6-month juice fasts and one 4-month juice fast.

Before Brother Air started his first fast, we had met Charles Lloyd after a Columbus concert. He knew that we were Ehretists and wanted us to convene with him after the show. Following a very deep conversation about Lloyd's fasting expeditions in the mountains of Europe and the regaining of his night-vision eyesight abilities, he demanded that we get him some music reflecting our lifestyle. This was a great inspiration for what would evolve into the Breathairean Ensemble.

So, tell me about your journeys on the island.

Peace, Love, and Breath!

-Spira

Raw Foodism in the Dominican Republic

Email sent by Cy on May 19 2008 at 5:12 pm

"One disease, long life; no disease, short life"
-Chinese medicinal proverb

and a quote that popped into my head upon reading your note, which I think speaks to some of what we and a lot of other natural food/earth lifestyle converts are doing.

"Phew!"" is my response to the last message you sent me. I am taken aback by your personal history and journey into a higher nutritional state and self. What an amazing, phenomenal dude you are! I've never come across anyone along your lines in my entire life, but I bet you get that a lot. Had to take a breather and process your message/massage a bit and chill out over the weekend. People have been getting shot over here and generally acting a fool with the presidential elections and pre-shenanigans and aftermath this weekend.

So the island...I'm here doing volunteer work and something of a personal journey/exploration of some of my roots. Quisqueya is where the turbulence of slavery/colonization decided to regurgitate my maternal side. I had only been here once as a child for a funeral, which is now a strange montage of palm trees, mosquito netting, and coffin wood to me so I'm trying to see/learn/understand/deconstruct/reconstruct more now.

Quisqueya is an interesting, one-of-a-kind island. On the positive end, it's gorgeous down here with a rich, vibrant, and productive land that generously outputs substances in direct alignment with my raw ways. I'm talking papayas and pineapples from outer space, foods from the heavens crashing down onto the land directly and literally. And nothing compares to reliable sunshine. It's also broadened my understanding of self and of my mother. I began a journey some years ago, sort of mapping out my heritage and the trajectories of my predecessors, and this is another stop. On the negative end, I think coming here with ideas about what Quisqueya/Dominican is much idealized in my head, I now realize sometimes clashes with what I see here, and painfully so. I have come across many sights and sounds that I seem to absorb more personally than a complete outsider. Things like rampant materialism, stagnant poverty, gender dynamics, and most of all race relations, either get under my skin or incite shell construction. The rampant materialism and the stagnant poverty go hand in hand. Much of this is rooted in the constant contact Dominicans have with their relatives in Nueva York. There are about 8 million Dominicans/Haitians living on the Dominican side of the island and about a million Dominicans living in the States. And what do you think are the #1 and #2 sources of revenue for the island? Sadly, remissions and tourism. The internal economy here is truly a mess with an elite class hogging everything and poor people galore, many who claim to be middle class but definitely not by US standards of middle classdom. Already problematic enough, the constant contact with US culture (or faulty, gaudy projections of it) leads to material expectations that are severely misaligned with people's earning capacity and skew decision-making about feeling good today versus bettering tomorrow. So, for example, you'll see a family of seven living in a wooden, tin-roofed bungalow with a cable satellite attached to the roof. Or people with spruced-up Hondas with mega speakers (always with the mega speakers here!) with no money to buy food for their kids. Still another example is one of my friends who makes $120 a month as a receptionist and has no problem spending $40 on a bottle of perfume. Truly, the people I see working hard are the people who come here or are born here but with origins in Haiti. So with Haiti, you get this extremely complicated and racially stratified relationship.

Getting back to the positive though, I am privileged to be here. It's hard at times—there's no water and no electricity sometimes and I'm living on a serious budget like I haven't had to for many years—but it's taught me so much about myself, about simplicity, and the idiosyncrasies of Dominican Spanish. I've encountered many positive energies and (re-)discovered jewels within myself that I might have overlooked in the grind of Nueva York. I live in a small city of about 80,000 called Mao (Taino for "land between rivers") up in the northwest, in a province called Valverde. I'm working with a special-education school doing teacher training and parent capacitation work, as well as teaching a sexual health curriculum with a local youth group. I'm hoping to add some REAL nutrition education in the mix in the Fall. I plan on staying here about 10 more months and then returning to the States.

Being raw here is wacky as living on Mercury. But people already think I'm strange, so adding raw foodism to the mix is no big deal. Sharing food here is huge. A lot of times people express their love or care for you by sending you "food" (ironic because it's usually a death substance). So I try to share as many fruits and vegetables as I can and let people know up front what I eat. I think it is far ruder to reinforce deadly eating habits than to politely refuse to eat something that I am offered. The food culture here is pretty different than in the States. Being an island, Quisqueya lacks the global reach that most urban centers in the United States have with regard to accessing a wide variety of foods; and even when items do get imported, they are costly, out of reach to the majority here. Most people here eat variations of the same thing every day: rice, beans, a meat dish (chicken/beef/pork or goat usually), and sometimes a vegetable (a simple iceberg lettuce salad, cooked okra, eggplant, or platano are common) with garlic, onion, and a lot of salt thrown into almost everything.

Overall, I find the Standard Dominican Diet to be a half-step up from the Standard American Diet (S.A.D.) because most people have a 2-hour lunch/siesta when they can come home and make their food. People don't care much here for fast/instant food and take pride in preparing their own food; and at least meat and eggs here, for the most part, aren't hormone- and chemical-laden and factory created. However, there are some major culprits in the Dominican diet which seem almost inescapable because they would require a radical restructuring of the food culture to change. Mainly the mountains of white rice people eat daily and other processed starchy products like pasta and bread that looks like Styrofoam; and to me, even more deleterious, the preponderance of white sugar. The concept of juice here, which shouldn't really be called juice but that's how it is here, usually means squeezing or extracting liquid from a fruit, mixing it with water and sugar, and drinking it. I think "sin azucar" has been the most useful expression for me in this country. It all reflects in the health problems people have: diabetes, hypertension, midsection obesity, and more. Vegetarianism isn't unheard of but it still gets jaw dropping reactions. Mostly in the capital, you'll find vegetarian restaurants (some brought by Hindu nomads). But raw-food-wise, I'm basically on my own.

So that's the island for you in a nutshell. I'm happy to be in communication with you. I see we are striving towards the same thing, to open people's eyes to the truth of their own radiance through pure foods intended for human consumption, bodily cleansing, and natural living, and that is a wonderful thing!

As always it's a pleasure hearing from you and writing to you. Connect and share again when you have the time and will.

Paz, amor, libertad, poesia, Cy

Preparing for a Juice Cleanse

Email from Cy on Friday, August 1, 2008, 9:41 AM

Peace to you, Spira,

Hoping this reaches you in a state of supreme well-being. I wanted to thank you for writing back, for taking the time to read my poem, and also for the package that seems to be on its way. I'm looking forward to picking it up in the capital (si Dios quiere) in 2 weeks, where it will hopefully be waiting for me.

You use a lot of colors in your poem and I see a runaway rainbow quality of your stage landscape as well. What does color mean to you, and what colors do you radiate?

My mom's visit was good, fun, wacky, and stressful. We're quite star-crossed in our personalities but we managed to have some learning experiences exploring Santiago and relaxation time in Puerto Plata. The sound of the ocean crashing is aural therapy to me.

I'm feeling like I'm approaching ready to do a juice cleanse and I wanted to know if you had any energies or perspectives to share on this. I also wanted to ask you to elaborate on your perspectives about cayenne pepper/spicy substances. My experience is that it helps to break down and push mucus up or out. I first noticed this when I would make salsa and I would drink the juice remaining after the salsa was gone, which was just tomato-lemon and cayenne or jalapeno juice, and I've witnessed others use spice to alleviate coughs/chest colds along the same thinking. Other sources tell me it is damaging to the stomach lining and causes digestive trouble in general. And then I've read and probably most agree with the Ayurvedic notion that we have constitutions, therefore nullifying umbrella dietary rules.

Connect soon and continue to radiate timeless being of the upper dimensions,

Cy

Email Sent on Saturday, August 16, 2008 1:37 PM

Greetings Cy!

As always it is a privilege to connect with you. I am glad to hear that your mother's visit went well. I think that I understand what you mean when you say that the family meetings can be a bit stressful. I feel blessed to have a family that supports me regardless of my "radically extreme" lifestyle/philosophies, but the social relationships are difficult. With the knowledge that I have about the human body, it is hard to see my loved ones continue to dig their own graves with their teeth. I used to eat out with my aunt almost every day and when I stopped eating in restaurants, our relationship was made even more complicated. It is such a shame that the social interaction of the mucus un-culture usually revolves around eating and the celebration of filth. The word *companion* even derives from the phrase "bread fellow," implying that the foundation of all friendly relationships is eating. I envision a community/society where breathing is the source of celebration and fasting is the norm.

Change of Skin Color on Diet

I do love to explore radiant colors in my poetry, especially shades of violet, which fit me very well. As an aspiring hue-man being, color means everything to me. One of the most profound discoveries of my physiological journey was to realize that the races of the world are nothing more than conditions made possible by pus and mucus. The longer that an individual's bloodline has been eating wrongly, the lighter the person is. Ehret, a white German from the 1800s, forcefully asserted this point. Needless to say, this caught my attention. He often mentioned how much darker he became while fasting and sunbathing. He remembers being mistaken for an Indian due to his new, dark, reddish-brown skin. At first, this just seemed like a radical philosophy; but I began to see similar things happen on my own body. As I started to clean myself, I became darker and darker. When I went back to eating mucus, I could see my skin become paler. Ultimately, no matter what hue we start with, as we eliminate the slime that permeates our body, we cannot help but to get darker and become the black holes[34] that we are meant to be: Blood + Oxygen − Mucus = Hue-Man.

Juice Fasting

I am very happy to hear about your juice fast. In response to your question about cayenne pepper and spicy substances (all types of vinegar can be thrown in too), I will say that they do nothing to help heal the body. This kind of pepper acts as an irritant and a stimulant that stirs up

---

34. For definition of "black hole," see page 284.

195

the waste that is already in the body. The patient may feel that mucus and toxemias are being extracted due to the effects of the stimulant, but irritating the tissue system is definitely not the most efficient way to bind and eliminate poisons from the body. This conclusion can be drawn from the simple fact that a clean body cannot ingest these poisonous materials. After my first 6-month juice fast, I had to let many of those irritating condiments go; but that was okay because my taste buds had moved on to the next stage. I am quite critical of the "master cleanses" that advocate cayenne pepper, syrup, etc. It is one thing to have an uncontrollable craving for these stimulants as you transition away from them, but they need not be interspersed with fasting on purpose. Nature appreciates rational simplicity, and less is always better. As a rule of thumb, I avoid mixing things as much as I can; and if I do not need it, I eliminate it.

The process that you described with your jalapeno juice could be compared to the suppressive properties of other kinds of poisons. When a new poison is introduced into the body, the body stops working on its current eliminatory task to deal with the new problem. This is what happens with many pharmaceutical drugs as well as herbal solutions. The patient smells or ingests something, and the condition feels changed temporarily. This additive approach does not help eliminate the real source and storehouse of the problem, which is the colon. If the patient were to be in the habit of doing enemas to combat uncomfortable nasal/lung/etc. eliminations while doing away with the mucus-causing foods, the ultimate cleansing process will be initiated and the days of the uncomfortable nasal liquid and physical pains are numbered.

The best thing to ingest to be more aggressive with the loosening process of mucus is lemon juice. When I was attempting to neutralize my flesh-poisoned body at the beginning of my transition, I would eat 2 or 3 lemons, rinds and all, every day. Now I do not do that because it would be too physiologically aggressive and counter-productive. In my opinion, the transition is not only a lifestyle but a high art, possibly the highest art before the science of breath. Ultimately, the goal is to cleanse with the least and most efficient substances—oxygen being number one, followed by fruit sugar, and then starchless vegetables.

Incorporating Lemon Enemas

My challenge to you would be to do your juice fast while experimenting with lemon enemas every day. The daily irrigation of the bowels will immediately advance your progress further than you could imagine. It may seem a bit extreme to do it every day at first but, as we now know, the eating of disease-producing foods is far more extreme, and our bodies need as much help as they can get to rectify a lifetime of ignoring the constitutions of our physiologies. Many people feel the need to brush their teeth every day or rub soap on the outside of their body, but the only reason the outside is so nasty is because the inside is incredibly filthy. Layers of pus and mucus permeate our tissue systems, and they can only be taken care of through a lifetime of consistent cleansing. To help put our condition into perspective, I will share one of Brother Air's experiences with you. Brother Air has practiced the transition diet for almost 30 years and has engaged in many extended, raw fruit-juice fasts. During a recent 9-month fast, he described a long and horrifying piece of mucoid plaque that came out in his enema. He has been doing enemas for 30 years, been mucusless for years, and he is still eliminating chunks of mucoid plaque. I have had a similar experience, being into a long period of no solid food and eliminating 12-inch long, mozzarella-cheese-looking strands of odiferous mucus. After all of this, I stopped asking why I need to do enemas every day and started to ask how many times a day can I do them.

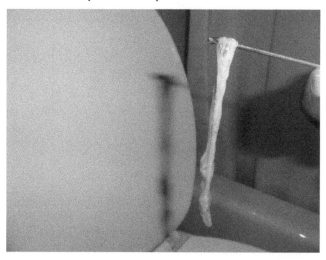

Mucoid Plaque (from Spira)

197

Let me know how your cleanse goes and feel free to send me more of your music/poetry/writings/etc. I look forward to hearing from you soon.

Peace, Love, and Breath!

Prof. Spira

Importance of Breaking the Fast Properly

Email sent by Cy on Friday, September 5, 2008, 11:34 AM

Spira,

The juice cleanse is going well. I haven't gotten around to the enema or "lemena," if you'll have it, yet, though I have been putting lemon in my drinking water as an experiment of an idea I came across recently and it seems to be having a positive cleansing effect on both the water (making it living) and me.

What are your thoughts on nutrition/the body-mind state and relationships? I don´t mean just romantic-type relationships but all human interchanges. I am finding myself hesitant to hang with a lot of people because I anticipate the debauchery that is the everyday norm: beer-drinking, pizza-eating just to name a few examples.

xoxo,

Cy

Email sent by Spira on Monday, September 29, 2008 3:35 AM

Greetings Cy!

Brother Air and Breaking a Fast Properly

I hope that everything is going well with you and your cleanse. I have actually been juice fasting for the past 3 weeks and am now moving into some liquid days juxtaposed with fruit days. Many fasting instructions, including Ehret's, have the faster break a long fast with a big meal of fruits or vegetables, but I have found it much more effective to transition in and out of different levels of fasting. I really learned this lesson when I saw Brother Air break a 9½-month fast by eating a piece of watermelon. During his fast, he gave off a vibration of perfection and had an unbelievable Midas touch. I have actually never seen anything quite like it and am still in awe of this phenomenon, which we call "the magic." It got to the point where Brother Air would have free drum equipment show up at his house along with boxes of lemons and free pineapple juice. However, once he broke his fast, insanity ensued. I remember a scene a few days after he broke the fast where he was buskering at an outdoor market called Findley Market, where he was attracting some very strange vibes. In fact, Brother Air had to reprimand

199

one crazy woman who was dancing around him, touching him, and rolling her eyes; and one man almost got beat down for annoying him.

The reason that Brother Air broke his fast was so that he could do it on his son's Earthday, which is very noble. I am not quite as noble yet and I tirelessly attempt to allow my physiological condition to dictate my transition. For instance, I always say that my first long fast had more to do with me allowing my body to do what it wanted to do. I had to do the hard mental work of eliminating the impediments of a debilitating socialization, i.e., being "too skinny," or I "gotta eat," etc. All of this mythology swam around in my head, but I did not allow it to affect my experiment, which was to find out if the body is an air-gas engine. If it was not, I would have died; but if the body was an air-gas engine, as it is, then what we call a fast is the rule and eating is the morbid exception. Then why do we eat? We are either doing one of two things: adding to our internal cesspool or helping our body loosen and eliminate the unnecessary dross.

Columbus

The past couple of weeks have been deep. Right after I moved to Columbus, my electricity went out for 4 days and both of my computers were ruined. On top of all that, my car broke down. When this kind of thing goes on, I know that I need to fast through it. I have found that when I fast through the hard times (when it would be customary to indulge in some heavy food drugs), it makes the average times much easier. We are now in the second week of classes and I am enjoying them so far.

The Fallacy of Nutrition

Question: What are your thoughts on nutrition/the body-mind state and relationships? I don´t mean just romantic-type relationships but all human interchanges. I am finding myself hesitant to hang with a lot of people because I anticipate the debauchery that is the everyday norm: beer-drinking, pizza-eating just to name a few examples.

At first, I interpreted your question wrongly. I have great contempt for the word *nutrition* due to its erroneous implications and sadistic history (see Antoine Lavoisier, François Magendie, and Mulder). The term presupposes that the body needs to intake and assimilate elements that are burned away or lost. We call this the additive principle or the belief that the body needs something to be a body. This belief system allows its followers to rationalize eating unnecessary and debilitating substances. Which substances are necessary and which are unnecessary, and why? For me, the word is irreconcilable. It could be argued that the term refers to that which nurtures or sustains us, but air is the only substance that does this, regardless of what we do or do not eat. Of all of the erroneous concepts handed down through antiquity, our concept of nutrition is the worst. It is critical that we begin to change the language, and the term *nutrition* has been found guilty and is on the chopping block. I do not mean to come across too harshly, but the word is responsible for so much misunderstanding and death that a severe thrashing is warranted.

Dealing with Social Relationships on the Diet

Our physiological condition will greatly influence whom we have relationships with and why. I did not realize how vital eating is to our social makeup until I began to stop. At first, I could still hang out with my old friends and date females who were not into their health. But at some point I become more and more repulsed by the debauchery. Here I was doing all of this work to stay alive and I was surrounded by folks who played beer pong. Luckily, Cincinnati was the place to be and I was able to join a small yet strong community of like-minded people. This was a key for me. I was able to see how much faster I could develop with the support of a community. My relationships with people outside of this community became more business-oriented and formal with the style of Dale Carnegie as an inspiration. This is one reason why I have been able to deal with academia. I am great with formal interactions, but when everyone drops their formality and heads to Starbucks, I head for my enema bag. When people want to go have coffee or lunch, I just tell them that I do not eat in restaurants, which of course leads to more discussion. I do, however, keep the discussion light and respectful. I know that if someone really wants to know what I do ,they will not be able to hold back their questions; so I keep these discussions as simple as possible (but I am always planting seeds that may blossom years down the road). I have found it to be much more effective to tell people the details of what I do after they have known me for a while (like a year or two). This way, they cannot put up an invisible shield when I am unleashing truth in their direction. When the time is right, I then invite them into my world of fresh juice and fruit away from their bars and grills. This way they can see for themselves that a transitional lifestyle of fruits and vegetables is not as crazy as they think it is.

One of the most amazing things that I have experienced during my transition is that whenever I truly let go of past attachments/addictions (e.g., hanging out at dance clubs/bars, going to loud parties where I would instigate fights, eating in restaurants, etc.), something else would come to fill the void. I learned that if I was ever going to be able to help my friends and loved ones, I needed to get myself together, which meant spending time away from them outside of their direct emotional influences.

Eating Out is Like Going to a Crack House

I explained it to some of my old friends who felt hurt that I would no longer go out to eat with them: Imagine that I had a friend named Tom. We had been best friends since elementary school and we used to do everything together. At some point Tom started to do crack cocaine. I still love my friend Tom, but I do not feel comfortable going with him to the crack house to watch him get high and kill himself. The point is that we should not put ourselves into environments that are not conducive to our lifestyle because we want to hold onto a certain kind of social interaction or friendship. Since I have gotten over that hump, my friends and family have a great respect for what I do, and the adversarial and "misery loves company" attitudes have disappeared. If I would have confronted the adversarialism head on, it would have greatly impeded my progress, and I will not let anything that I control do that.

In sum, it is completely rational for you to feel repulsed by the lifestyles of those who are killing themselves with impunity. It works on both sides of the equation; you feel repulsed by their actions and they feel uncomfortable because you are not taking part in the reindeer games. What emerges is an inequitable relationship that $700 billion couldn't help. It would be great if we had the power to save our friends and family from slow suicide, but this cannot be possible until we heal ourselves and unite as a community. The legitimacy that accompanies human solidarity is one of the most influential tools for social change and it is definitely needed when you are trying to sell the hardest product that there is to sell, which is health.

I look forward to hearing from you!

Peace, Love and Breath!

Spira

Email sent by Cy on Friday, October 17, 2008 12:39 AM

Hola Spira,

Hoping this reaches you in wellness. I wanted to first thank you again profusely for the media you sent me. I have finally gone through all of it (except a planned rereading of the Ehret book you sent) and I enjoyed all thoroughly. I got to better know your perspectives through your radio show broadcasts, and the music is divine. The fasting suite (www.bit.ly/brother-air-album) that your friend Brother Air did especially sounds of freedom to me. Some of the other works remind me of Pharoah Sanders and the way he hops around and juxtaposes concepts. What else did I want to say? Ah, I wanted to tell you that your transformation is one of the most remarkable I've seen. Your before and after look like two different people almost entirely, except the eyes.

Things are going well on my end. My mental patterns are migrating over to my return with increased strength every day. I'm not necessarily rushing to get back but I want to return in the right way in certain aspects. A lot of things in my life are up in the air and my mind keeps shifting between a state of returning to NY where I lived before I came here versus broadening my viewpoint to consider other places. My head is going Mercury to Pluto and back, so it's a little commotive. I did a headstand today, though, and that made me feel better.

Cy's Fast-Breaking Techniques

My juice cleanse is going well. It's like no other I've been through, but I suppose every cleanse has its quirks and bits. I'm on Day 21 right now and planning on going until Day 26. My juice regimen has been pretty simple. Mostly I've been doing pineapples, apples, parsley, spinach, cantaloupe, papaya, and lots and lots of oranges because they are the fast fruit that can be hand-juiced when the power goes out here (country folk with no electricity, I have heard, employ innovative techniques in juicing, hand grinding and so forth, but I'm not yet adept at such things). I use a less sweet variety of oranges that people normally add sugar to >:(but which I find pleasantly sweet and sour on their own.

I agree with your point that fast breaking should be gradual. My body necessitates it. Anytime I've jumped straight to solid food from juice cleansing, even something as small as a handful of grapes, my body rejects it and throws it right up. I have to go through blended liquids

203

inclusive of pulp first and then slowly get back to pure solids over a few days. I read something (which I'll attach for you) about juice cleansing that suggested soaking prunes in water overnight and drinking the liquid and eating the prunes, and that the first foods one should intake after a juice cleanse should be purely eliminative to maximize the benefit of the cleanse. That's what I'm aiming for this time.

Your technique of cleansing during tough times, literally keeping things moving, is dope and noted and makes perfect sense. Stress collects in the system, so this approach is like a stress anti-glue. Thanks also for your words on social interchanges versus food-drink intake, let's say, since you disfavor the word nutrition. I would tell you it's pretty deep here, but just as a means of being sarcastic to emphasize the wackiness of some of the people I've come across. I'm nobody's judge, honestly, until it comes to people stepping into my domain, in which I am highly discriminatory. Every invite or social session that crosses my path, though, seems to be mixed in with heavy indulgences in what I call non-food substances disguised as foods, alcohol, cigarette smoking, and conversations of the type I don't want to be involved in.

Though the DR is a far cry from the bustling live-food resources and people that span Nueva York, I am happy to have met my first raw-food friend in the DR, a former volunteer who decided to live here after she finished service, so I'm looking forward to building with her.

Spira, you are funny. I am not a brilliant educator. I just like to read a lot and love learning as much as I can. I'm sort of insatiable, so I'm always looking for more, trying to get beyond. All I can say is, I hope to radiate more every day.

You be well, keep breathing and living the genius that you are, brave warrior.

Cy

Long-Term Healing with an All-Fruit Diet

Email from Cy on Wednesday, December 14, 2011 11:14 PM

Professor Spira

Hey brother Spira, I appreciate the resources you sent me and will be going through them one by one. Seriously—major thanks to you for this!

Apparently and sadly, the fast-food restaurant in hospitals is not something new: http://bit.ly/nytimes-fast-food-hospital

On another topic, what's the deal with people in your old stomping ground or at the person who did this?: http://bit.ly/whites-only-sign-at-pool

To end it on a positive, you might be interested in checking out a webinar this Sunday hosted by Dr. Gabriel Cousens (whom I think I've spoken to you about). He'll be talking about scientific insights on fructose and glucose.

Peace/love/health/radiance as always,

Cy

Email from Prof. Spira January 6, 2012

Cy!

I definitely find the issue of healing with a fruitarian diet versus vegetables to be very important. Modern raw-foodist camps seem to be drawn around this issue. Some, such as Cousins and Hippocrates, emphasize vegetables, while Doug Graham is a bit more on the fruitarian side. I remember when you wrote the following about your experiences with sweet fruits versus sub-acids:

> The taste of sweet is fine but the effects on my system are unbalancing and it makes me physically and mentally unstable. So when people tell me fruitarianism is the way, I could see it with non-sweet fruits like tomatoes and peppers, but I focus more on a general low-glycemic raw intake, which includes vegetables of a wide variety, sprouted beans, seeds, nuts, sprouts, cold-pressed oils, less sweet fruits and modest intake of a few sweeter fruits on occasion. I love fruit and believe it's necessary but I have to watch it with that, and the foods that

make me feel the most balanced are vegetables, kale probably taking a top position.

The Question of Fruitarianism

I checked out Cousins' video on his perspective about simple versus complex sugars. I had also read some of his books a couple of years ago when you initially recommended them. I've also gotten to know a young lady in Columbus who studied with him and has instituted local, raw-outreach events. Although I appreciate his success in fostering interest in higher levels of dietary consciousness, I vigorously disagree with his views on the role of fruit in human diets and its role in healing. Fundamentally, the construction of his dietetic paradigm is based upon allopathic Western medical thinking of chemical isolationism and nutrition. I find no value in the measurement of calories, fats, or protein. For me, the beauty of chemistry is to observe the perfection of nature as the omnipotent laboratory.

It should be mentioned that I also fundamentally disagree with the "fruitarians" that he speaks of. Most of the modern fruitarian gurus I've come across are also coming from an allopathic perspective, talking about where their protein comes from. Also, most are not mucus-free fruitarians, as they consume a lot of nuts, seeds, and avocados. I do not advocate this sense of fruitarianism at all. I find the works of early fruitarian thinkers such as Hilton Hotema, Fry, Heyward Carrington, and Arnold Ehret to be much more enlightening. (Many such authors have full books featured here www.soilandearth.org.) In general, I'm troubled that the work of many modern diet gurus do not reflect the advanced lifestyles and thinking of the natural-hygienic/back-to-nature movement Hippy Roots (visit www.bit.ly/hippie-roots). If there is an aspect of European culture to be put on a pedestal, it would be the "back-to-nature" consciousness. However, they could only take it so far.

When raw gurus or otherwise fear or avoid fruit, it is often an expression of their own physical toxicity. Since proper nutrition is often their focus, when they begin to experience neurological symptoms when eating fruit, they still blame the fruit. Either the fruit is too depleted or humans shouldn't eat too much of it. This is what meat eaters often do. Stop eating meat, get sick and scared, eat meat again and feel fine. One-sided vegetable rawists eat fruit and experience thyroid and diabetic symptoms. Why? It is because of the toxicity inside the person who ate the fruit. But instead of fasting through the foggy brain and weakness to regenerate, they propose a vegetable program where most fruits are eliminated. For a S.A.D. eater, this should give relief; but, the endocrine glands will not fully heal at that vegetable level. I must emphasize that the symptoms of elimination are real, but their cause and method of healing have been grievously misunderstood. Overall, humans need to shift their manic obsession with a wrong concept of nutrition to a focus on the constitutional toxic encumbrances of the body. When we put this into perspective, we will begin to understand how long it will take to eliminate and transform back into full-fledged, fruit-living humans.

The paradigm that Ehret's work has fostered is one of transition. Fundamentally, at its most rigorous, it was and can be used aggressively to heal people on their deathbeds. As a lifestyle, the transitional principles and methods may be adapted to any person to slowly and safely transition to higher states of dietetic excellence. If a person's goal is to get off of mucus and cooked foods, then that may be achieved. If someone wants to sustain fruitarianism, then this may be done. But the higher a person wants to go, the longer it will take and the harder he or she will need to work. I do believe that humans are fundamentally a frugivorous species. Then why can't we eat only fruit now? It is almost unfathomable to grasp the enormity of our level of degeneration. Through generations of wrong eating, we have saturated our organisms with a level of putridity that cannot be described in language. Thus, the physiologic karmic debt that one must pay when one decides to pursue this path back home is rough. At different points of the journey, people will go through periods of healing crises, or "falls," where any number of symptoms (including those from diabetes, thyroid issues, etc.) are full blown and possible for an extended period of time.

In any case, people are not experiencing symptoms from the fruit, but from the toxic waste that is in the body/bloodstream. Measuring all of the calories and fructose in the world cannot help a person who has a toxic bloodstream and constipated lymphatic system. This, then, should be the subject of intense focus and consideration. If we could take our obsession with nutrition and put it into the toxic "obstructions" that are in our constitution from birth, we could get much further. What is the level of toxicity in the body, and what is the most efficient way to use food to clean it out? Once cleansed, in time, the cells of the body can regenerate any disease.

Spira's Fall

But this method takes much more time than most people care to spend. In July, I passed out, which initiated an intense healing crisis. We call this "the fall," and it is usually had by all who fervently pursue this path. Fundamentally, it is a total rewiring of the body's electric system (endocrine). I experienced every symptom described by people with diabetes, thyroid, and other conditions. When I ate fruit, I experienced foggy brain or felt faint. I had intense anxiety from when I got up to when I went to bed, and nothing, fruit, vegetable, nor mucus could quell the feeling. I tried exercise, which did not help. However, doing a million sit-ups would later help put off panic attacks. Although I had prepared myself for this moment for 9 years, I was still terrified. Few have made it to this part of the path, and fewer have written about it. I can always recognize someone who has had a similar experience and become scared of fruit. Many, like dietetic writer Stanley Bass, wrote against Ehret, after having tried "raw" or "fruit" lifestyles and fell on their face. If you take a closer look at what they did, most of these cases were from the sickest of sick people trying to just go raw or onto fruit with absolutely no transition. Twenty to 30 years of transition may have been necessary to do what they tried to do in a matter of months. (Ehret and Robert Morse are no exception: visit Morse's website at http://www.drmorsesherbalhealthclub.com/ .)

In the spirit of science and sociology, I decided to go to OSU medical doctors to go through their tests. I wanted to evaluate the process after having not seen a medical doctor for more than 9 years. Ehret conducted many private and public physiological experiments on himself to explore various areas of his dietetic perspective. I will write a detailed article on that experience one day, but overall it was a joke. I was almost unable to drive my car 10 miles to the clinic from intense anxiety attacks, and my time with the doctors resulted in iron and B-12 supplements, along with anxiety medicine I could take before "going to work." Of course, this was only after several visits. Epic fail!

I knew that I would ultimately have to dig deeper than I ever had to pull myself out the situation. I had tried all levels of short-term fasting and even back to mucus to find a way in. I realized this was going to take a lot of time. I spent a couple weeks clearing out as many of the stressors in my life as possible. I quit bands and told everyone I was off to work on my dissertation. Harder still was explaining to loved ones that I would not be speaking with them for weeks or months. Once I had dealt with the fundamental stressors of modern life, I began to lemon/water fast. I unplugged the phone and internet; did not talk with anyone. As I got into the fast, I descended to a level of weakness and fear on par with the ninth circle of Dante's Inferno. I thought to myself, "This is why people are so scared of this diet. I now understand why it is easier to die strapped to a bed with IVs than to confront this reality." I was so weak, I could not listen to music for several weeks. Eventually, I could tolerate classical music. After a week and a half of water fasting, I had some dry days. I then got into a serious grape cure consisting of freshly juiced grapes (all types) and grape eating. Overall, I navigated my way through various levels and types of fruit-based fasting and started to get my vitality back. The times that I ate a salad or green drinks, I could feel my detoxification come to a halt. Ultimately, it has taken 6 months of grape-juice fasting and berry eating to come out of my fall. As I gain my vitality back, I am able to compose and practice music for hours on end. I watched my body go through an amazing transformation (again) and I know for a fact that this level could not have been achieved with the intervention of many vegetables. Two days ago, I had my first salad in several months. It was a success and I am beginning to transition back into the world. Yet, after my experience of the past 6 months, I am thoroughly convinced that humans are 100 percent frugivorous.

Healing the Endocrine System

Yet, most people who suffer from chronic blood and endocrine issues would not consider a 2- to 6-month recovery time for their ailments. Plus, we are vigorously conditioned to avoid weakness; thus, to get weak before getting strong is deeply feared. Since we have trodden so far from nature, we still want to blame fruit for our weaknesses rather than the inherent toxicity of our ailing bodies. Over the past 6 months, I felt the capillaries in my brain being revitalized. I could feel a tingle in my feet as my parathyroid started to reactivate. I watched my pancreas turn back on and relearned how a human digests food. As my adrenal glands started to function, the anxieties went away. (I could handle and make Black music again!) As my kidneys started to filter lymph, I could see and smell a level of acid waste in my urine that I had never experienced before. As sulfur from 18 years of prescription drugs eliminated, I had painful gas and watched the dark orange and light blue rings around my irises change and subside. (*Note: I also took this opportunity to study and experiment with iridology, botanical/herbs, reflexology, acupuncture, and chiropractics. Self-directed psychotherapy, meditation, and prayer also played a significant role in this journey. I'll write about some of these things in the future.)

This is the first time I've ever written about any of this, and have only talked about it with one or two other people. My hope is that my experience can help to put the depth of our pathological condition into perspective. In the hustle and bustle of the modern world, 6 months to fast and heal in isolation is hard to understand. "He just needs to eat a cheeseburger and get back in the game," is what I heard one person say. It is unlikely that they would understand, but his sentiments are indicative of so many others in the Western World. Everyone seems to look for the right diet, pill, etc., to heal or suppress the symptoms. Since time immemorial, fasting has been the omnipotent cure for human illness. But, I observe that the conception of modern-day "time" has inhibited our path toward true health, possibly more than fasting. A lot of people are getting hip to fasting, but finding a way to understand the "time" of healing is difficult. What if a permanent cure could only be achieved by 6 months or a year of fasting and detoxing in a stress-free environment? Such a level of consciousness and understanding would result in a fundamental change in society. Provisions would be made at one's job while one went to eliminate. In the meantime, we must survive by any means necessary.

I've seen families that practice the diet band together in remarkable ways. In some cases, when one is down, fasting through an intense elimination, the other works to make money and support the family. Practicing this diet in these dark ages is like being at war, but the battle is often waged laying on one's back in bed. Needless to say, this war would not make a very entertaining video game.

Enjoy your vacation!

Peace, Love, and Breath!

Spira

Chapter 7—Advanced Analysis and Historical Inquiry Inspired by the Mucusless Diet

Leaders of the Physiological Revolution: A Short History

The following was originally posted on the Breathairean Ensemble's website, breathairmusic.com. It places Ehret's work, and our efforts, into a historical context.

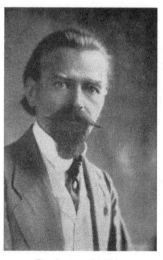

Prof. Arnold Ehret

A History—The late 1800s proved to be a remarkable time in the history of human health. In Europe, many philosophers and scientists began to question the conventional and formative concepts regarding the nature of the human body and the purpose of human existence. In the 1890s, a cultural renaissance inspired by the works of Nietzsche, Goethe, Hesse, and Baltzer emerged as pioneers began to experiment with natural cures, raw foods, vegetarianism, and social reform. Thousands of young Germans rejected urbanization to pursue a more natural lifestyle.[35]

---

35. Kennedy, Gordon and Kody Ryan, "Hippie Roots & the Perennial Subculture," Hippy.com, May 13, 2003.

In the early twentieth century, many Germans began to migrate. Countless members of the counter-culture relocated to southern California, where they could practice their natural lifestyles in a warm, comfortable climate amidst an abundant supply of fresh fruits. The lifestyles of the immigrants had a profound influence on many young Americans who adopted the natural beliefs and practices. In 1914, Professor Arnold Ehret, counter-culture icon and author of the *Mucusless Diet Healing System*, moved to southern California and began to operate a very successful sanitarium.[36] He published many works and established a school where he instructed students on how to administer the *Mucusless Diet* to patients. Before his tragic and untimely death, Ehret cured and educated thousands through his teachings and life example.

Throughout the mid 1900s, the counter-culture would inspire various social movements including the beatnik and hippie generations.[37] Although founded on the principles of a vegetarian lifestyle and a natural, physical culture, the pursuit of superior health began to decay into the experimentation and indulgence of unnatural stimulation. Despite the deterioration of the original ideals of the movement, Americans continued to read Ehret's literature; however, very few wholeheartedly subscribed to his teachings.

In the late 1970s, a group of African Americans in Cincinnati, OH began to experiment with Arnold Ehret's *Mucusless Diet Healing System*. Led by Victor Buttrom, these Ehretists forged ahead, endeavoring to maintain a mucusless lifestyle. In 1983, jazz drummer and percussionist Brother Air met Buttrom and began to pursue the *Mucusless Diet*. Over the next 25 years, Air would contribute much to the diet, especially in regard to its practice as a lifestyle. Air's adoption of the daily lemon enema, as well as the formation of his family around the *Mucusless Diet*, created a template for all Ehretists to follow.

Art and music have always played a major role in the promulgation of the *Mucusless Diet*. In fact, it reached the African Americans in Cincinnati through a music concert. Artists and musicians have traditionally been drawn to the possibilities of the *Mucusless Diet*, while others have preferred to ignore it. In November of 2003, Professor Spira and Brother Air traveled to see Ehretist and saxophonist Charles

---

36. Kennedy.

37. Kennedy and Ryan.

Lloyd. This meeting inspired Brother Air to engage in his first 8½-month juice fast. Also, Lloyd's insistence on hearing Air and Spira's music planted a seed for the creation of the Breathairean Ensemble.

In 2004, Spira and Air assembled a group of musicians to fulfill a series of engagements at the University of Cincinnati. Upon completion of the concerts, Professor Spira, Daktehu, "Uncle" Eddie Brookshire, Baby Babaji, and Brother Air continued to rehearse without a musical engagement in sight. Soon they realized that the band was vegetarian and Ehretist. It was then that the band became known as the Breathairean Ensemble, and it was established that the group would function as a support system for its members who are striving to achieve physiological liberation. The musicians endeavor to carry Ehret's torch through the twenty-first century and inspire all who are dedicated to self-preservation and the pursuit of eternal life.

Visit www.breathairmusic.com/physiological-liberation/.

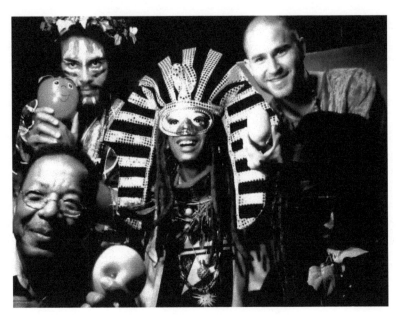

The Breathairean Ensemble

Prof. Spira: Trombone, Keyboard, Vocals

Uncle Eddie Brookshire: bass

Baby Babaji: Percussion, Flute

Daktehu: Saxophones

Brother Air: Drums, Percussion, Hand drum rig

Who is Brother Air?

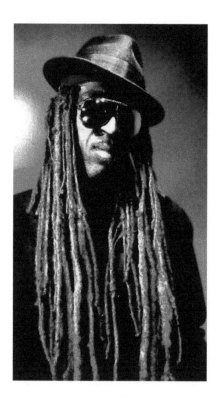

Biography

Meet the man that does not eat. No, seriously, since 2002 he has eaten for only 11 months while abstaining from solid food for over 49 months. Brother Air's life revolves around the practice of the Mucusless Diet Healing System, and he believes that there is nothing more important than the preservation and regeneration of his bloodstream. During his career, Air has traveled across the globe sharing countless musical experiences with the Universe and its many musicians, but today you will never see him perform in a bar. Frustrated with filthy bars and uncreative musicians, Air decided to take his art to the streets, where he developed his legendary Hand-drum Rig and famous V=P-O rhythm.

Brother Air was born and raised in Cincinnati, OH, where he began playing the drums at the age of four. During his teens, Air was profoundly inspired by civil rights activist and vegetarian Dick Gregory.

He then developed a serious attitude about health and began to study the human body and its diet. In the early 1980s, Air came into contact with a group of Cincinnatians that practiced Arnold Ehret's Mucusless Diet Healing System. He then became an Ehretist and committed his life to achieving physiological liberation through practicing the Mucusless Diet Healing System.

Since the 1980s, Air has contributed a great deal to the practice of the Mucusless Diet Healing System. In 1995, after 15 years of doing daily distilled water enemas, he began to administer lemon enemas multiple times a day. This remarkable action would set a new standard for all serious Mucusless Diet practitioners to follow. Then, in 2001, Air consumed nothing but fruit for an entire year, followed by a succession of three 100-day fasts. In November 2003, after a very inspirational meeting with jazz saxophonist and Ehretist Charles Lloyd, Air successfully embarked on his first 8½-month juice fast and completed a solo percussion album, entitled "Brother Air," to celebrate his success at the finale. He would then complete a 7½-month fast followed by a 9½-month fast, only eating for a few months in between. Air, who is a community activist and family man, has inspired a countless number of people to consider plant-based lifestyles by shattering the many erroneous myths regarding how the human body operates.

Today, Brother Air can be seen across the country buskering and sharing his passion for the Mucusless Diet with his son, Baby Babaji. Air's family was formed around the Mucusless Diet and is the blueprint for all families pursuing physiological liberation. Air's ultimate goal is to open a sanitarium to teach fasting, mucusless diet, and the importance of the lemon enema/colonic.

If you don't know how your body operates, you can be told anything.

-Brother Air

Watch rare footage of Brother Air talking about the Mucusless Diet and fasting:

9½-Month Fast: 30-Year Practitioner of Arnold Ehret's Mucusless Diet speaks! **(visit www.bit.ly/brother-air-talk)**

Peace, Love, and Breath!

-Prof. Spira

216

Critiques of Biological and Social Theory: Protein and Nutrition

The following is a paper that I wrote for my "Research Methods in African American and African Studies" graduate course at the Ohio State University. It is a critical response to a chapter within a book by Alan Garfinkel about social scientific theory, called *Forms of Explanation: Rethinking the Questions in Social Theory*. Although you could benefit from reading Garfinkel's chapter, it is not necessary to understand my arguments in this essay. Overall, I took the opportunity to examine and refute many of the most injurious Western dietetic principles within the context of a college paper. After its completion, I had the pleasure of presenting it in a lecture format to my class. Overall, I scored very high on this assignment and did very well in this class. I make mention of this only to empower you to step outside of the box and challenge yourself and others when you feel inspired to do so. Conventional wisdom might suggest that it is not prudent to include such information or make such controversial arguments in a college essay. But if the arguments are strong and the reasoning sound, those trained in critical reasoning may be inclined to respect your work.

A Review of Garfinkel's *Forms of Explanation, Rethinking the Questions in Social Theory*, Chapter 4 Biology and Society

In this chapter, Alan Garfinkel continues to examine the theory of logical explanation by arguing against the use of "individualist" methods of reasoning within the biological sciences and social theory. To do this, he examines a number of biological theories that have shaped social theory. He strives to expose possible fallacies caused by suppressed presuppositions imbedded within individualistic theories by offering structural explanations that focus on macro processes. Garfinkel's method not only illuminates the big picture, but allows for more effective individualistic inquiries. He makes a strong case for the need of structural explanations that illuminate macro processes and he demonstrates the problematic nature of reductive and individualistic reasoning. Although he attempts to make structural arguments that are free of concealed presuppositions, he manages to commit the fallacy himself. In the following review, I will examine an explanatory frame proposed by Garfinkel and strive to uncover problematic presuppositions within his argument.

Garfinkel asserts that social structures are radically underdetermined by individual differences. Therefore, biological explanations, whose paradigm is inherently reductive, can never fully explain social structures. He asserts that the explanatory frame:

biology → society

suppresses and presupposes the social structure, and that a more effective explanation would be

biology X society → society[38]

Garfinkel then supports his claim with an example from standard genetic theory—where the suppression of environmental factors is quite evident. Phenylketomuria (PKU) is a genetic disorder where the body is unable to utilize the amino acid Phenylalanine. Essentially, the enzyme that converts phenylalanine to the amino acid tyrosine is deficient, and chemicals from other enzyme routes accumulate in the blood and body tissues. If left untreated, the patient may suffer from vomiting, irritability, rashes, foul-smelling urine, microcephaly (small head), prominent cheeks, upper jaw bones with widely spaced teeth, poor development of tooth enamel, and decreased body growth. However, most of the symptoms of the disease are avoidable through newborn screening, diagnosis, and dietary management.[39]

Garfinkel points out that because the symptoms primarily derive from the patient's inability to metabolize phenylalanine, a diet that is free of the enzyme would create the most favorable postnatal environment. The standard treatment for the disorder consists of a diet that avoids foods rich with protein, such as meat, fish, poultry, eggs, cheese, milk, dried beans, and peas. Instead, measured amounts of cereals, starches, fruits, and vegetables are recommended.[40] In other words, Garfinkel's proposition is that a vegan diet free of albuminous foods will create a dietary environment where the patient will not suffer the effects of PKU. Albumin is a water-soluble protein found in egg white, blood plasma, and milk. Therefore, Garfinkel asserts that the effects of the

---

.38 Garfinkel, Alan, *Forms of Explanation: Rethinking the Questions in Social Theory* (New Haven: Yale, 1981), 116.

39. Kerr, D. MD and Ms. J. McConnell, *Living with PKU* (Inherited Metabolic Diseases Clinic, University of Colorado Health Sciences Center, Denver, Colorado, 1991), accessed November 8, 2008 http://www.medhelp.org /lib/pku.htm.

40. Garfinkel, 117.

disease cannot be explained by genetics alone and offers an explanatory frame that illustrates a double dependency on two environments:

genetics X womb environment → trait T (inability to metabolize enzyme)

and

trait T X normal diet → PKU[41]

What is a Normal Diet?—It is plain to see that the effects of PKU depend upon the dietary environment of the patient. However, the problem with Garfinkel's argument is that he fails to define what a "normal diet" is. He presupposes that a normal diet is one that contains phenylalanine (i.e., meat, fish, poultry, eggs, cheese, and milk). It is quite problematic to assume that a "normal diet" includes these foods, when a large segment of the world's population does not consume them. Many of the world's peoples show long histories of vegetarian lifestyles, including people of India and Asia. In fact, Dr. Miriam Lowenberg writes in her book *Food and Man*, "There are and always were more herbivorous people, the next most prevalent being the carnivore, followed by the omnivore."[42] If Lowenberg's assertion is correct, then a vegetarian lifestyle free of foods containing phenylalanine is more "normal" than a carnivorous or omnivorous one.

It is not clear if Garfinkel presupposes a carnivorous or an omnivorous diet to be normal. Given the diversity of dietary habits possessed by the peoples of the world, what is a normal diet? It is generally believed that people within the United States and Europe are omnivorous, but this presupposition ignores the wide range of dietary practices found throughout the world. This assumption may stem from the belief held by Western medical and dietetic theory that protein-rich foods are vital for human subsistence. The proponents of this theoretical structure often claim that diets lacking in protein are in some way primitive or inferior. The problem with this paradigmatic view is that many of the world's people have subsisted well on diets free of protein-rich foods.

---

41. Garfinkel, 117.

42. Lowenberg, Miriam E., E. Neige Todnunter, Eva D. Wilson, and Moira C. Feeney, *Food and Man*, 2nd ed. (New York: John Wiley & Sons, 1974), 3.

Given that the intake of protein is vital for the human organism to live, how is it possible for people to subsist on diets that have little or no protein in them? How could children diagnosed with PKU survive on a diet that is protein deficient? It is reasonable to assert that if protein-rich foods were absolutely vital for the subsistence of the human being, then it would be impossible for any human to live without them. The case can be made that Garfinkel is using the term "normal" to identify people who conform to Western dietetic theories of protein consumption and nutrition. Garfinkel's aim is to show the problematic nature of structural presuppositions, although by presupposing "normal diets" to be ones that conform to Western dietary standards he falls victim to the same reductive trap that he is arguing against. Nevertheless, another interpretation of the word "normal" suggests something that is healthy and natural. This explanation would introduce an even greater structural problem and raise questions about what is truly necessary for human subsistence.

For now, let's assume that a normal diet is a healthy and natural one that provides what the body needs to survive. Given the wide range of dietary practices in the world, can it be determined what foods the human body biologically "needs"? First, let's examine the protein theory. In the early nineteenth century, a French physician and teacher of physiology named Francois Magendie conducted research on dogs in an attempt to find what food substances are essential. Lowenberg explains:

> When he fed dogs single foods such as sugar and water or olive oil and water, the animals died. Magendie concluded that animals needed nitrogen in the diet. He knew that both body tissues and many foods contained nitrogen, and he suggested that the nitrogen of the tissues **probably** [emphasis mine] came from food. The nitrogen-containing foods were called albuminous foods.[43]

Twenty-two years later, in 1838 the Dutch chemist Mulder gave the name *protein* to the nitrogen-containing material in albuminous foods. The word protein comes from the Greek word meaning first; therefore, the word itself presupposes that the first principle to life is albuminous foods (i.e., meat, poultry, fish, eggs, dairy, etc.).

This theory is problematic for several reasons. First, to presuppose that albuminous foods are the foundation for life ignores Lowenberg's

---

43. Lowenberg et al., 171.

claim that the world has always possessed more herbivorous people than omnivorous.[44] If protein is really the first principle of life, no human would be able to live without it. Second, it is self-evident that the foundation of life as we know it is breathing air. So the question remains, given that breathing air is essential for human life, and eating albuminous foods is not, what does the human need to consume?

In the late nineteenth and early twentieth centuries, a surge of medical researchers whose evidence challenged the newly developed theories of protein and albuminous foods emerged. In his book entitled *Fundamentals and Requirements of Health and Disease*, Dr. Thomas Powell MD challenges what he calls the "Nitrogenous Food Theory":

> This theory has enjoyed a long season of popularity and yet it is an undeniable fact that the notion that nitrogen is the prime essential of food is wholly fallacious, having no other foundation than an erroneous supposition and a misinterpretation of facts—errors which have led to a desperate misuse or abuse of the most valuable of all foods.[45]

He goes on to challenge the germ theory and asserts that albuminous foods play the most important role in most human illness. Finally, he explains that the vital machine of the living organism "owes its every movement, whether feeble or powerful, normal or abnormal, to the EXPANSIVE ENERGY OF CARBON DIOXIDE."[46]

Professor Arnold Ehret also stood against the developing theories of protein and nutrition. In his dietetic treatise entitled the *Mucusless Diet Healing System,* he asserts that albuminous foods, or as he calls them "mucus-forming foods," are the foundational cause of most human illness. He says:

---

44. Lowenberg et al, 171.

45. Powell, Thomas, *Fundamentals and Requirements of Health and Disease* (Los Angeles: Powell Publishing, 1909), 41.

46. Powell, 145.

Every sick person has a more or less mucus-clogged system, such mucus being derived from undigested and uneliminated, unnatural food substances, accumulated from childhood on.[47]

After having identified mucus-forming foods (albuminous foods) as the foundation for disease, he suggests that a mucus-free diet of starchless fruits and vegetables should be the goal of all true seekers of health. Furthermore, Ehret identifies the body as an air-gas engine whose primary need is air.[48]

To test this theory, Ehret effectively conducted many fasting cures on his patients and diligently took note of the astonishing healing potentials. He also experimented on himself by subsisting on extended fruit diets and long periods of fasting. Notably, he completed a series of public fasts monitored by government officials in Europe, with the longest being 49 days with no food or water. He concluded that it is more difficult for a pathologically sick body, one encumbered with pus and mucus, to fast (subsist without solid food) than it is for a body that has been cleansed with mucus-free foods for an extended period of time. Essentially, Ehret claims that the cleaner and healthier the body is, the less food it needs to survive.

How was Ehret able to subsist on fruit for years at a time and do month-long fasts? Given that protein is a vital part of the normal diet, why did Ehret not suffer from the symptoms of protein deficiency? According to much of the standard literature within Western dietetic theory, a human being should not be able to fast longer than about 14 days, not to mention have the ability to demonstrate great feats of physical and mental strength at its conclusion as Ehret often did. (For pictorial documentation of Ehret's physical changes during his experiments, please see Ehret 2001, 96-116.) Furthermore, an argument could be made that Ehret and his followers suffer from some sort of unprecedented eating disorder. A generally accepted definition of an eating disorder is a compulsion for, or avoidance of, eating that adversely affects the patient's physical and mental health. The question is, How were Ehret and his patients able to successfully complete long fasts and subsist on a mucus-free diet while improving their physical and

---

47. Ehret, *MDHS* 1924, 25.

48. Ehret, *MDHS*, 51.

mental health? [For Ehret's response to this question, please see Ehret, *MDHS* 1924)]

The protein-deprived dogs in Magendie's experiment may shed some light on this question. As stated above, Magendie asserts that the lack of nitrogenous foods led to the untimely demise of the dogs. However, Ehret offers a dissenting explanation about why the fasting dogs in Magendie's experiment died. You will recall Ehret's conclusion that a body free of mucus and toxemias can live for longer periods of time without the intake of solid foods. Given that Magendie's dogs had a diet of mucus-forming/albuminous foods before the fasting experiments, it is fair to say that they had a mucus-clogged system. The question now becomes, Granted that the dogs suffered from mucus constipation, were they clean enough to fast without loosening up a fatal amount of internal waste? Ehret would argue that they did not starve, in the Western sense of the concept, but that they drowned in their own dross.

Ehret's findings led him to believe that fasting helps loosen mucus and toxemias within the body, but he warns people who are too encumbered with waste against engaging in long fasts. Essentially, Ehret believed that true starvation occurs when the blood can no longer be oxidized due to a morbid amount of waste within the bloodstream. It is paramount to understand that Ehret only prescribes fasting within the context of his system of eating; that is, the eating of mucusless foods interspersed with occasional fasts.[49]

It is plain to see that the structural presuppositions found within Western dietetic theory need to be reconsidered from the root level. Therefore, given that a "normal" diet is a natural and healthy one, it is not possible to define this kind of eating habit within the paradigm of Western dietary theory. Since Magendie's interpretation of nitrogenous substances in the nineteenth century, an extremely sophisticated scientific infrastructure has developed to support the protein theory; but, it appears that the core of this premise is quite erroneous. I would argue that Western medical science is no closer to determining what a truly "normal" (healthy and natural) human diet is than Socrates was in the fourth century BC.[1] The problem is this: Given the power and

---

49. Ehret, Arnold and Fred S. Hirsch, *Rational Fasting for Physical, Mental, and Spiritual Rejuvenation* (Beaumont, CA: Ehret Literature Pub. Co., 1965).

influence of the Western medical establishment, many people, including Garfinkel, take its structural presuppositions for granted.

Given the proposed explanatory frame above, to what extent can it help explain the issue of dietary habits? Can this structural frame be applicable to different social environments? Given that this new explanatory frame works in the United States, will it also work in China, Bali, Venice, and Ghana? The question now becomes, What social environments have phenylalanine-containing diets? Above, I argue that diverse social environments have different dietary norms. Consequently, in order for Garfinkel's notion to help explain dietary habits and deride structural presuppositions, a "normal diet" would have to be one that contains phenylalanine:

Phenylalanine = Normal Diet.

Given the social formation of dietary norms, are there any societies or groups of people who subsist on diets that are free of phenylalanine? Many of the world's peoples show long histories of dietary habits that are deficient in phenylalanine, including people of India and Asia. In fact, Dr. Miriam Lowenberg writes in her book *Food and Man* that "there are and always were more herbivorous people, the next most prevalent being the carnivore, followed by the omnivore."[50] Herbivorous diets do not usually contain phenylalanine. In light of the above, it is probable that there are societies that have dietary habits that are free of phenylalanine-containing foods.

Considering the range of dietary practices around the world, the interpretations of what constitutes a "normal" diet is extraordinarily relative. It is possible that many vegetarians, vegans, raw foodists, fruitarians, breathairean practitioners, Ehretists, macrobiotitians, rice dietitians, Atkins dietitians, flesh eaters, as well as the practitioners of the so-called Standard American Diet (S.A.D.) believe that their dietary practices are "normal." To avoid the fallacy of the existence of "normal diets," perhaps the label "albuminous diets" or "phenylalanine [mucus]-containing diets" would be more useful and effective for Garfinkel's explanatory frame:

genetics X womb environment → trait T (inability to metabolize enzyme)

and

---

50. Lowenberg et al., 3.

trait T X "phenylalanine containing diet [mucus]" → **PKU**.

At this juncture, it is possible for the following question to be raised: To what extent are phenylalanine-containing diets more prevalent than non-phenylalanine-containing diets? This question would speak to the potential "normalness" of Garfinkel's assertion. The argument here is that if the majority of the world's peoples have diets that contain phenylalanine, then it is logical to use the term "normal diet" within Garfinkel's explanatory frame. This argument illuminates the following issue: Can it be assumed that the majority of the world's diets contain phenylalanine without collecting data to support the claim? Given that there is data that suggests that the majority of the world's peoples have diets containing phenylalanine, to what extent would this help explain why some societies do not have phenylalanine-rich diets? The problem with the above line of questioning is that it suppresses the social formation of normal dietary practices. If Garfinkel's notion of "normal diets" is meant to be relative to the social environment that created them, then the possible prevalence of phenylalanine-containing diets is not pertinent.

In sum, it appears that Garfinkel's notion of "normal diet" may not work given the diversity of dietary habits around the world. Garfinkel asserts that phenylalanine-containing diets are necessary for PKU while offering the following macro level explanatory frame:

genetics X womb environment → **trait T (inability to metabolize enzyme)**

and

trait T X normal diet → **PKU**.

Garfinkel's explanatory frame appears to suggest that a "normal diet" is one that contains phenylalanine. If social interactions solidify dietary norms, this would propose that phenylalanine-containing diets are normal within all societies. This proves to be problematic because phenylalanine-rich diets are not normal to all of the world's societies. It can be argued that phenylalanine-containing diets are prevalent among world populations, therefore making it normal; but if "normal diets" imply a dietary habit that is relative to individual social environments, then the aforementioned prevalence is irrelevant.

Note

¹ In Plato's Republic, Socrates discusses what kind of a diet is best for the inhabitants of their republic. While Socrates first suggests a meager diet with fruits, etc., Glaucon argues for a diet that will produce what Socrates calls a "city of pigs." Socrates explains that an indulgent diet, consequently filled with plenty of albuminous foods, will ultimately result in the necessity of more physicians being employed. My question is, Given that the chosen dietary lifestyle would undoubtedly produce more sickness, why did they decide to permit it within their republic?[51]

---

51. Warmington, Eric and Philip G. Rouse, eds., *Great Dialogues of Plato*, Book II, W.H.D. Rouse, trans. (New York: Mentor, 1984), 169-170.

Iron and Blood: Lesson One

Posted to Facebook in 2009

I am creating lessons that open up discussions about commonly held interpretations within the fields of physics and dietetics. As a result of Arnold Ehret's work and the physiological research conducted in Cincinnati over the past 35 years, a new and important paradigm has formed to explain and understand physical phenomena. The problem is that very few health seekers outside of the United States have been exposed to its theories and explanations. My aim is to use Ehret's assertions and our new knowledge of the human body to examine the usefulness of currently held interpretations of natural phenomena. Consequently, we will develop better explanations and deepen our understanding of Ehret's work.

The purpose of this lesson is to philosophically analyze the nature of human blood through Ehret's theoretical frame.

View the following Video: Why Iron Kills Stars: Black Hole Birth (visit www.bit.ly/black-hole-iron)

As you watch the video, meditate on the nature of human blood and consider its iron content. In what ways can you connect the nature of human "iron" to the radioactive iron found in space, i.e., the sun and other stars? What happens to the iron in your blood when it combines with oxygen? What happens when oxygen comes into contact with iron mined from the Earth? To what extent can explanations of these questions allow for a deeper understanding about the potentials of our physiology and the nature of our blood?

I wrote the following poem a few years ago. Read it before and after watching the video. You may also want to watch the video a few times. Can you find anything problematic with our contemporary interpretation of what a black hole is?

Red Blood Vessels

Before death
When the earth had no water
I breathed freely.

Radioactive red suns flowed
Through my veins
Illuminating the heavens.

I was the glowing black hole,
Host of the Omniverse,
Chosen to settle among
Blood red pines and tend

Abundant pink and purple
Phalaenopsis with my exhale.
Vibrant petals stretch and bloom.
Masterfully knitted with great detail.

The dark green stems tunnel down
Bringing forth the smell of
Love and the sound of Bliss.

The suns in my Omniversal vessels
Flowed freely, stirring the eternal flame
Emitting the vibrations of cleanliness,

OOM BOOM BA BOOM, Bloom the
Effervesce of the immortal host.

Before the ravishing of ripe red apples
And tart scarlet cherries was a time
Of pure music. Love the style, Air the
Harmony, Hue the melody, Man the
Instrument and OOM BOOM BA
BOOM the driving rhythm.

-Professor Spira

Please review "The New Physiology, Cont." Lessons VIII-IX, Blood Composition and Blood Building in the *Mucusless Diet Healing System*. Also, examine some definitions for "Radioactivity." Use the following questions as a platform for further discussion.

Questions

1. Some people say that health is about the radioactivity of the blood. What is meant by this?

2. What does Ehret think "white blood corpuscles" are?

3. Who is Dr. Thomas Powell, and what does he call mucus?

4. Who is Julius Hensel, and what is his argument regarding the composition of human blood?

5. Fill in the blanks: "I presume that the truth and importance is this: The _____ color of blood is the most characteristic quality of this "quite special sap" and is due to _____-_____, _____." -Arnold Ehret, *Mucusless Diet*, Lesson VIII.

6. In Lesson IX, Ehret argues that his dietary system will help build perfect human blood. Explain how and why.

What are White Corpuscles?: Lesson Two

c. 2007

How can it be understood with certainty that white blood cells are in fact waste: decayed, undigested unusable food substances as proposed by Professor Arnold Ehret? The process by which we "understand" or "know" something is quite complex. An epistemic approach would force the question, How do we know what we know? Can we acquire such knowledge through experience and observation? Can we obtain it through rational thought? Or is our "knowledge" merely a socially constructed belief system? The important issue here is the extent to which Ehret's thesis on blood composition is useful. My argument is that Ehret's hypothesis is quite relevant. However, for the reader to discover its significance, a close examination of Ehret's proposition is necessary. In this paper, I will 1) examine Ehret's arguments about blood composition, and 2) review the historical and dialectical emergence of the white blood corpuscle theory.

Ehret claims that the Western notion of metabolism, or the "science of the change of matter," is the most absurd and dangerous doctrine-teaching ever imposed on mankind (Ehret *MDHS*, Lesson VI). He explains that it has helped spawn the fallacious "additive principle." The additive principle is the belief that certain food substances must be consumed to nurture the body and replace used-up cells. Here, Ehret does not accept the additive premise and argues that energy and body revitalization does not derive from the intake of food. Rather, energy (vitality) is determined by the physiological cleanliness of a waste-free body. Consequently, the only purpose for eating is to aid the body in eliminating waste. In other words, the cleaner the body is, the less food it will need to consume and the more vitality it will emit. Ehret explains, "Claiming that you must replace cells (which are not used up as you can plainly see), with high-protein food from a cadaver, partly decomposed meat, and which has gone through a most destructive heat process of cooking! The fact is that you accumulate more or less of the wastes in your system in the shape of mucus and its poisons as the slowly growing foundations of your disease and the ultimate cause of your death." Given the above, where does this accumulated waste go? Does it ferment and rot in the intestines? What happens if this waste is not eliminated in a timely manner? Is some of the waste incorporated into the tissue system? How does the waste accumulation affect the bloodstream?

Ehret begins to address the above in Lesson VIII. He writes, "The problem is this: Are the white corpuscles living cells of vital importance to protect and maintain life, to destroy germs of disease, and to immunize the body against fever, infection, etc., as the standard doctrines of physiology and pathology teach? Or are they just the opposite—waste, decayed, undigested, unusable food substances, mucus, pathogen, as Dr. Thos. Powell calls them? Indigestible by the human body, unnatural, and therefore not assimilated at all?" (Ehret *MDHS*, Lesson VIII). Ehret argues that what has been labeled "white blood" is nothing more than uneliminated waste. He supports his claim with the following observations: 1) pathology asserts that "white corpuscles" are increased in case of disease, and 2) physiology claims that they increase during digestion in the healthy body and that they derive from high-protein foods. Thus, high-protein foods, or mucus-forming foods, are involved in the creation and perpetuation of white corpuscles. Nevertheless, how do we know that these corpuscles are not agents for good in the body? More importantly, why has medical "science" embraced and promulgated the theory that white blood is normal?

Given the pathological condition of our bodies, it is possible that white corpuscles were originally viewed as normal due to their prevalence. The proposition is this: Since white corpuscles are so common, they must have a function. Ehret argues that white corpuscles do not help protect the body from predators, but are actually dead material. He explains that the skin pores of man are "constipated by white, dry mucus" and that his entire tissue system is filled-up and filled-out with it (Ehret *MDHS*, Lesson VIII). In other words, dead waste materials are being wrongly viewed as living blood cells. To support his claim, he provides observations of his own experiences. "Everybody knows that an extreme case of paleness is a 'bad sign.' When I appeared with my friend in a public air bath, after having lived for several months on a mucusless diet with sunbaths, we looked like Indians and people believed that we belonged to another race. This condition was doubtless due to the great amount of red blood corpuscles and the great lack of white blood corpuscles. I can notice a trace of pale in my complexion the morning after eating one piece of bread" (Ehret *MDHS*, Lesson VIII). Why does Ehret become darker after being on a mucusless diet with sunbaths? Why does his complexion become pale after eating bread? Ehret's anecdote implies the following: The tissue system and bloodstream of the human body is permeated with waste materials.

These waste materials (i.e., mucus and pus) cause the body to reflect light. The more waste that the body contains, the more reflective it becomes. Consequently, the color of man is dependent upon the quantity of mucus within him. Therefore, the physical distinctions that we describe as "race" are nothing more than physiological conditions of pathology.

To understand the above, it is important to know the role of iron in the blood. When iron that is mined from the earth comes into contact with oxygen, dark rust is produced (iron oxide). When our blood iron comes into contact with air (i.e., oxygen) it also rusts. Clean blood that is free of white corpuscles easily rusts when oxidized. To demonstrate this argument, Ehret tells of his experiments with self-inflicted bleeding. He found that when he ate a mucusless diet for an extended period of time, a knife wound would heal immediately with no secretion of pus and mucus. He would also suffer no pain or inflammation. Thus, the oxygen would mix with the iron in the blood and rust immediately. However, when he ate mucus-forming foods, his wounds did not easily heal and he suffered from pain. He also became paler. This experiment suggests that 1) a mucusless diet promotes clean blood, 2) clean blood is free of white waste materials, and 3) clean blood becomes dark when oxidized. My question is this: Given that blood becomes dark when mixed with oxygen on the outside of the body, to what extend does this happen inside the body? When clean blood is oxidized through the act of breathing, does it rust and darken? Hensel's argument may shed some light on these questions. "In our blood, albumen is a combination of sugar-stuff and iron oxide, but not to be found or recognized (discovered) in such a way that neither the sugar nor the iron can be found by ordinary chemical tests. The blood albumen must be burned first to make the test perfect" (Ehret summarizing Hensel's "Life," *MDHS* Lesson VIII; Hensel and Schindler 1967). Consequently, the red color of blood is due to iron oxide, i.e., rust. Furthermore, the ability for red blood to become oxidized is dependent upon the absence of albumen (i.e., mucus/waste).

In his scientific treatise on physiology entitled *Fundamentals of Health and Disease*, Thomas Powell explains, "The biologic, physiologic, and much of the dietetic and pathological teaching of this day and age is founded upon the assumptions that the "white blood corpuscle" is a "living cell"; that it is "differentiated" into the tissues of the body; that it is a "phagocyte" or germ-devourer; and that the material in which it is

232

found and from which it is formed . . . is the 'physical basis of life'."[52] He then asks the following question:

> Is it not entirely reasonable to suppose that the motility of the white blood corpuscle is due to the forces, not of life, but of death; to the processes not of vital duplication, but of chemical dissolution—that is, to the combined effects of chemotaxis, disintegration and gaseous expansion . . . ?[53]

Powell's argument parallels Ehret's by asserting that the leukocyte (white corpuscle) is "not a living cell, but a particle of dead and perishable material."[54] He adds that "the irony of the situation into which the leukocytic addendum to the cell theory has led us is not only perfectly discernible, but as cruel and relentless as the grave, since it is to the effect that the more 'tissue-building' material (white corpuscles) the sick man carries in his circulation, that more pronounced is his debility and emaciation, and that the more 'vigilant policeman' (phagocytes) he has to guard and defend him, that more certain and speedy is his destruction."[55] Let us now shift our attention to the historical and dialectical emergence of the white corpuscle theory. My guiding questions are as follows: what is the origin of the white corpuscle theory and why early scientists viewed these corpuscles as "living cells." My aim is to provide a broad overview of the emergence of the theory. As a result of technological advances in Europe, simple and complex microscopes appeared in the sixteenth and seventeenth centuries. In 1656, Frenchman Pierre Borel, physician-in-ordinary to King Louis XIV and credited with being the first to use the microscope in medicine, described a type of "worm" found in human blood. In 1657, Athanasius Kircher, a Jesuit priest and scientist from Germany, examined blood from plague victims and described "worms" of plague. In 1661, 1664, and 1665, blood cells were observed and discerned by Marcello Malpighi. Also, after dissecting a black Ethiopian, he asserted that black

---

52. Powell, 263.

53. Powell, 275

54. Powell, 292.

55. For further reading, see Powell, "The Cell Theory," 263-294.

pigment was caused by a layer of mucus just beneath the skin.[56] In 1678, red blood corpuscles were described by Jan Swammerdam of Amsterdam, a Dutch naturalist and physician. The first complete account of the red cells was made by Anthony van Leeuwenhoek of Delft in the last quarter of the seventeenth century. A more thorough examination of the scientists and their interpretations mentioned above is forthcoming in a future essay.

By the nineteenth century, scientists had varying theories about the nature of blood cells. Powell explains that there was a major controversy about what the corpuscles should be named. Some suggested "colorless corpuscles," as the leukocytes were then called, and others preferred pus corpuscles. The father of the cell theory, Prof. Rudolph Virchow explained, "Under all circumstances, this layer resembles pus in appearance, and since, as we have already seen, the colorless blood cells individually are constituted like pus corpuscles, you see that we are liable not only in the case of a healthy person to take colorless blood cells for pus corpuscles, but still more so in pathological conditions when the blood or other parts are full of these elements."[57] Powell goes on to claim that the supposition of the "white blood corpuscle" as a living organism is the result in part by the "lifelike activities that it displays at a certain stage of its existence."[58] Here, the reader must be reminded that technological advancements often do not produce better explanations. Given the ability to view blood on the cellular level, some scientists concluded that the colorless cells were disease-causing waste materials, while others believed that they were life-saving agents. Powell points out that many of his colleagues had an affinity toward the latter.

In sum, Ehret was not alone in claiming that the colorless material in blood is dead waste. It is of the utmost importance that we begin to seriously consider the implications of what Ehret terms the "wrong cell theory." Far too many people have needlessly suffered and died as a result of the dead corpuscle fallacy. We must stop using the erroneous reference "white blood corpuscle." The term blood presupposes that it

56. Klaus, Sidney, "A History of the Science of Pigmentation" (Blackwell Publishing.com, 2006). www.bit.ly/pigmentation-history, accessed February 8, 2007.

57. Powell, 268.

58. Powell, 270.

is a living cell. I propose that we refer to the material as dead corpuscles or white waste. Virchow's "pus corpuscle" may even be a viable option. One of the reasons that it is important to understand the above is because it has a direct influence on how we think about our dietary system. Understanding this fallacy will help true health seekers put their condition into the proper perspective. Once it is understood that pus corpuscles are waste, then we can begin to ask very important questions regarding our dietary practices: Given that white corpuscles are waste derived from pus- and mucus-forming foods, how can they safety be eliminated from the bloodstream? What is the nature of blood that is cleansed of white waste materials? What is the significance of grape sugar and how can it help form perfect human blood? These questions will move us to Lesson IX on Blood Building.

The Question of Breathaireanism

Posted on March 24, 2006 by Root to the Ehret Club Forum:

Question: "Breathaireanism. Ok, I'm down with that theory BUT . . . if man originally was to live on air, were animals not? There are some animals that haven't changed in millions of years. So they are still in the unchanged original Creator's form, right? They still eat. In fact, don't all animals take in food and water in some form? And they eat mucus-forming food, too. They still have the desire to eat and search for food. Soooooooooooo, when you read things that Wiley Brooks says, you have to wonder. Any thoughts?" -Root

Posted on March 24, 2006 by Professor Spira:

As Ehret points out, the human body is an air-gas engine that runs on oxygen. I realize how hard it is for people in our condition to understand this without truly living it. We are in such a morbid situation that it is hard for us to fathom going a year without food, much less existing without food and drink all together. I did not begin to truly realize that I was an air-gas engine until I witnessed a man effortlessly fast for 8½ months. There was still doubt until I investigated myself by fasting for 6 months. As always, I am not saying that people need to be trying to achieve these kinds of fasts now, I would much rather hear about people learning to become consistent with their transitions and enemas. Ehret does not recommend long fasts for most practitioners. Brother Air is an incredibly advanced practitioner and a true pioneer of these higher levels of fasting. At this point, striving to become mucusless for a decade or two is more important than trying to complete long fasts or do a strict fruit diet with a body that is not clean enough to endure it. There are no shortcuts. So many people try to skip over the transition only to encounter terrible falls that scare them away from Ehret forever. It is important to try to use your logical thinking to trace your way back to a breathairean level. If you can fast for a day, then it is possible to fast for a week, then a year, and so on. But this level of fasting will come naturally as the body gets cleaner and cleaner.

In regard to your questions about animals, they are also air-gas engines. Just as we have to find the proper comfortable transition for our individual conditions, each species represents a different degree of mucus poisoning. In fact, the implication of the Mucus Theory uncovers the embryonic secrets to the development of all of the different races and animals. It is now plain to see why it is absolutely absurd to believe that we evolved from animals when it may have been the other way around. As Brother Air explains, animals are nothing more than *undeveloped humans*—organisms that were unable to develop into a human being due to the constraints of their own mucus poisoning. Ernest Haeckel's *Evolution of Man, Parts 1 and 2* is an excellent resource to study how every living being on this earth goes through the exact same embryonic cycle. On your journey to becoming human again, you first went through a cycle that looks like a leaf, then a fish phase, cat phase, and so on until you got to where you are now. There is no biological cycle in existence that is beyond that of a human being. Everything in the universe is trying to become you. What if there was some obstruction in the way of your embryonic development? Literally, if you ate like a cat, you would be a cat. If you ate the proper amount of mucus to hinder your development at the dog stage, there you would be. The phrase, "you are what you eat" is not just some esoteric ideal to be brushed aside or laughed at, but it truly is the law. If you eat dead animals and dead substances, you will become a dead animal; but if you eat live produce, you will be productive. I feel that it is an absolute privilege to have the opportunity to reverse my crEATure-like ways. As we can see from nature, if we do not use our free will to stop eating the wrong kind of foods, Mother Nature will take over. Before they became fruitarians again, gorillas were avid meat eaters. But nature slowly transitioned them back towards humanness. The same is true of cows and horses, which are now vegetarian. All of these animals are going through their unique modes of eliminations to become clean enough to one day rejoin humanity. Yet many humans are eating in a way that will ultimately result in becoming fish and maggots. Indeed, all life is sacred; yet I have no desire to descend into these lower levels of existence if I do not have to. Once humans rediscover their true humanity as air-eating frugivores, they will be able to assist these undeveloped humans to higher planes of existence. As humans evolve spiritually and physiologically, the whole world benefits.

It takes many lifetimes and a lot of mucus for a human to degenerate down into the animal kingdom. Many of the ancient bones that they find, such as Lucy, were really humans on their transition down to the animal kingdom. Basically, if you were to take the theory of evolution and reverse it, you would have a more logical perspective on the degenerative cycles of the human. For a deeper understanding, you must study the embryonic phases of a human from the zygote (fertilized egg) to birth. You will see how every living organism passes through the similar phases until it reaches its ultimate potential destination, i.e., a human. Medical science erroneously asserts that the yolk sac is giving the developing embryo nutrition, when it is more likely providing the embryo with the right amount of mucus obstruction being passed down from the parents. In light of the above, every tree, leaf, flower, maggot, and chimp is trying to complete the cycle to become a perfectly clean human being. In every case, obstruction from the waste of uneliminated, constitutional encumbrances is the cause for the embryo's inability to finish the process.

In regard to race, Ehret proposes that skin color reflects the degree to which someone's body is or is not saturated with wastes (mucus). The taxonomy of race as we know it is a socially invented construct and not true physiological science. Today, most biologists concede this fact, but for years the concept of race was used to institutionalize a racial caste system where it was believed that "non-whites" were inferior to "whites." Yet, modern concepts of race did not exist 500 years ago. I know of no people who are as dark as black soil or as white as freshly painted white walls. *Melanin* is yet another erroneous and misunderstood concept. Brother Air often asks people who believe in this theory to extract some melanin from their veins. It's hard to get melanin or water out of our body, but we do have a "special sap" that we call *blood*. It would follow that we reexamine the nature of blood through Ehret's new physiological perspective. When we bleed, and the iron in our blood comes into contact with the air (oxygen), what color does it turn? If it is clean, it will turn black or rusty brown. The cleaner the blood is, the more quickly it clots, serves to heal wounds, and darkens. Thus, the more encumbered one's bloodstream is with pus and mucus, the harder it is to heal simple cuts through this process of oxygenation. Further, one's "hue" is nothing more than a reflection of one's physiological condition. Ehret, after long periods of fruit fasting, notes how he could see his skin color become paler after eating mucus-forming foods. "I can notice a trace of pale in my complexion the morning after eating one piece of bread." Ehret explains that the cleaner he became, the darker he got. Eventually, he became so dark that people began to identify him as an Indian.[59] I had a similar experience during my extended periods of fruit eating and juice fasting. My skin became very soft and several

---

59. Ehret, *MDHS* 1994, 72.

shades darker the longer I abstained from mucus-forming foods—even during the winter, when I had no access to sun.

As far as the people who claim to be breathaireans, like Wiley Brooks and Jasmuheen, these people come across to me as charlatans. They talk a good game, but do not practice what they preach. I have a perspective on what fruitarians and long-term fasters should look like, and these people do not exemplify this. It is apparent that these people have studied a great deal of the available mythologies surrounding a breathairean existence; but ask them about their transitions, or better yet, what they ate today, and you may be surprised. As Wiley tried to explain in one of his interviews, he eats McDonald's quarter pounders to stay in tune with his environment and the universe, while Jasmuheen tries to tell people that they can just stop eating and attain a breathairean level in a few weeks. I could turn you on to numerous books that talk about the implications of breathaireanism and the type of things that these individuals studied, but most of these books were not written by modern people who are true breathaireans. In fact, one of the reasons that I spell *breathairean* differently than the original *breatharian* or *breathertarian* is because I do not identify my understanding of the concept to be in line with most of its popular proponents. The mythological stories of breathaireans and immortals are found throughout folklore and ancient texts but they are myths only, because we do not have the proper physiological understanding to deduce a rational judgment from the information. At this point, it is of the utmost importance to continue studying the system. The breathairean level is not merely something to think about psychologically, philosophically, or mythically, but it is something that you will feel, experience, and know for yourself if you stay consistent with the *Mucusless Diet Healing System*.

Peace, Love, and Breath!

-Professor Spira

Chapter 8—Where to Go from Here

Final Thoughts

Over the past several years, there has been a tremendous surge in consciousness surrounding issues of health. There is a newfound desire among many to seek out cleaner, more sustainable, plant-based ways of living. Veganism, raw foodism, and fruitarianism are all terms that more and more people are using to identify their dietetic aspirations and lifestyle changes. Often made fun of for his gluttonous appetite, former President of the United States Bill Clinton has greatly improved his health by endeavoring to transition to a plant-based, vegan diet. Regardless of one's opinion about his politics, it is significant for a person with his public influence to not be afraid to be outspoken about his plant-based experiences—as the subject has traditionally been viewed as taboo among politicians and celebrities. With that said, an increased number of celebrities and athletes are also becoming more vocal in their support of plant-based lifestyles, colon therapy as a form of regular hygiene, activism against animal cruelty, and transitioning "off the grid" to cleaner forms of energy. The reality is that people all around the world respect and idolize many of these public figures and are being influenced to view plant-based realities with more consideration and esteem.

With that said, the world needs to be exposed to the tenets of the *Mucusless Diet Healing System*. Gluts of plant-based books, websites, and new dietetic gurus have emerged to promote health. The problem is that most of these books and gurus do not incorporate a mucus-free perspective or advocate a rational transitional system. Also, most attempt to articulate programs based upon a faulty paradigm of

241

metabolism, nutrition, and dietetics. Calorie myths, vitamin theories, protein fantasies, B-12 supplementation, probiotics, recommended restriction of fruit eating, misuse of herbal remedies, and so forth can be found throughout the plant-based, holistic, and naturopathic movements. Although some of the more advanced diet gurus praise Ehret's writings, it is often primarily for his innovations in the area of fasting and the short-term healing of thousands of terminally ill patients. Few have had the courage to truly confront Ehret's propositions about the "tragedy of nutrition," fallacies of metabolism, Mucus Theory, the formula of life (i.e., Vitality = Power - Obstruction), and Ehret's perspectives on the proliferation of various skin colors (race). Even fewer have attempted to incorporate Ehret's transition as a lifestyle.

I emphasize a slow, safe, incremental "transitional lifestyle" toward raw and mucus-free foods based upon the principles in the *Mucusless Diet*. I have yet to see a long-term "raw food" or fruitarian lifestyle program that offers and promotes an effective transition system. Transition is hardly even talked about by the most famous modern raw educators. Further, many of today's popular raw, vegan, vegetarian, and fruitarian diet programs have their practitioners eating a lot of mucus-formers (nuts, etc.) with questionable combinations and mixtures that only bring them back to sickness.

What do people do after their initial period of mucusless detoxification? Some people will want to go back to their old ways. Yet some want to find a way to live cleaner for a longer period of time. What should young people do who are interested in going raw/mucusless but not sure what to tell friends and family? For people who do not want to fall back into old habits or begin a cleansing lifestyle in an environment with challenging social pressures, it is important to not only consider the mechanics of Ehret's dietary system, but also the social implications. Personally, I have had the privilege of helping many people who could not stay on "raw" or "mucus-free" find a comfortable way to transition toward these states in a more permanent manner. I have also worked with many health seekers coming from a Standard American Diet (S.A.D.), and it is a thrill to see them learn of this information and make a commitment to physiological liberation.

Do your best in whatever situation you find yourself—I began the diet while in college and I had to learn how to deal with hard social issues. There were no online raw communities yet, and very few people around to support a plant-based lifestyle. I had no choice but to face these challenges alone. In the college dorm cafeteria, I would take heads of lettuce and greens from the salad bar that were only meant for display, and ask for extra lemons and better fruit. My efforts actually helped to get the cafeteria to offer vegan options and a better variety of produce. When I would go through the line, people often looked at me as if I was crazy. I learned how to explain what I was doing in a clear and simple way that allowed them to understand and kept them from verbally attacking me. My intention is to love everybody unconditionally, and I do not like unnecessary confrontation. Yet, in the beginning, I had a lot of meat eaters want to pick on me for eating fruits and vegetables. Confronting these kinds of social issues was very challenging, but I managed to navigate through them. Yet, I have seen far too many with the honest desire to practice the *Mucusless Diet* be derailed by the social dynamics of their environment.

My question is how can everyday people get into the transition and sustain it? First, I encourage slow, systematic lifestyle changes. I have seen my advice and personal experiences help many people learn how to change their lifestyle and thinking toward a mucusless existence. Mucuslessness is not just about diet, but a lifestyle and paradigm shift toward a worldview more in tune with nature. Second, it is important to study the resources that are available about the *Mucusless Diet* (see mucusfreelife.com). Here, I must note how important my time with Brother Air was. He has mastered the ability to practice the mucusless diet in an adversarial, stimulant-based reality. He did not run to practice the diet as a hermit in the mountains, but remained in Cincinnati, OH among his family and friends. In doing so, he learned not only how to practice the *Mucusless Diet* on its highest level, but how to do it in very challenging circumstances. From Brother Air, I learned that the art of the transition is not only about knowing what foods to eat but how to live a life of mucusless transition in the modern world.

Much of the advice I find myself sharing in conversations about the *Mucusless Diet* are about coping with the realities of practicing the diet, especially on a long-term basis. Most people fear becoming an outcast to their social segments or families. My hope is that some of the interactions that I've had with fellow health seekers in this book will aid you in your journey toward superior health. I also hope that my personal stories, historical analysis, and mucusless-based philosophical inquiry will inspire, empower, and edify you about what it takes to sustain a lifestyle of mucusless transition.

It is a large part of my life's work to help others transition toward a mucusless existence. A mucus-free people is a fundamental solution for many of the maladies afflicting the world today: human illness, pollution, depletion and misuse of the earth's resources, starvation, sanitation issues, impediments to spiritual evolution, and so on. We must find our way back to Nature or we will continue to suffer dearly for abandoning her.

Heal the World

Make it a better Place
For you and for me and
The Entire Human Race
There are people dying
If you care enough for the living
Make a better place for you and for me

-Michael Jackson

In order to heal the world, we must first heal ourselves. It is time for humans to rise up from our long slumber and return home to Mother Nature. It is time to choose life over death and calm peacefulness over drunken stimulation. Free yourself from the cave of constipation and be a beacon of light for others who desire freedom. Physiological freedom is at hand. Dispense with a culture of death and embrace a reality of life, free from the treacherous impediments of mucus eating. Imagine a world free of pain and suffering, sickness and disease. Take a breath and give thanks for the opportunity to cleanse, heal, and liberate yourself from physiological tyranny.

What would the world be like without mucus and pus eating?

Let's find out together!

Peace, Love, and Breath!

-Prof. Spira

244

Chapter 9—Breathairean Poetry

By Prof. Spira

"This will give an outline of the serious nature of my work and the necessity for your help in carrying it through as the greatest deed you can perform, upon which depends not only your future destiny, but that of a suffering, unhappy mankind on the verge of a physical and mental collapse."

-Prof. Arnold Ehret

$$V = P - O$$

Our bodies are Blueprints of the Universe
Vitality equals Power minus Obstruction is the Key

to

Immortality

-Prof. Spira

Red Blood Vessels

Before death
When the Earth had no water
I breathed freely.
Radioactive red suns flowed
Through my veins
Illuminating the heavens.

I was the glowing black hole,
Host of the Omniverse,
Chosen to settle among
Blood red pines and tend
Abundant pink and purple
Phalaenopsis with my exhale.

Vibrant petals stretch and bloom.
Masterfully knitted with great detail.
The dark green stems tunnel down
Bringing forth the smell of
Love and the sound of Bliss

The suns in my Omniversal vessels
Flowed freely, stirring the eternal flame
Emitting the vibrations of cleanliness,
OOM BOOM BA BOOM, Bloom the
Effervesce of the immortal host.

Before the ravishing of ripe red apples
And tart scarlet cherries was a time
Of pure music. Love the style, Air the
Harmony, Hue the melody, Man the
Instrument and OOM BOOM BA
BOOM the driving rhythm.

Fable of Aireater

Let me tell you a story about a time long, long ago
before death and destruction ruled the land.
A time before man knew about pain and suffering,
sickness and disease. There lived a people. A perfect
immortal people. People that had radioactive blood
coursing through their veins. I am talking about the
Breathaireans. I am talking about the Children of the Sun.

Among these children there lived one little boy named
Aireater who was blessed with the gift of song. Everything
that he looked at or touched burst out with joyous song.
One day Aireater was singing a beautiful melody and the
vibrations came out of his mouth and penetrated the earth,
creating a garden full of nothing but black grapes. Aireater
had never seen such a sight. For some strange reason he
was compelled to eat one of the grapes. And as soon as
he did he passed out and
slept for 50,000 years.

When he woke up he was totally confused.
He was in pain!
His skin was pale and wrinkly.
His hair was straight.
He had lost all of his powers,
except for one.
He still had the gift of song.
So he sung out:
"Children of the Sun, what have I done?"
And as soon as he did,
the children appeared
before him and told him
to stop eating. . . FAST!

Just like Aireater
we have forgotten
who we are and where
we come from. So we
must use our gift of song
to ask the Children of the Sun
for help.

Children of the Sun

Help me call upon the Children of the Sun
to see if they will grace us with their presence!
Clap your hands to the beat and repeat after me;

Children
Children of the Sun
Children, please tell us
What have we done?

Please Children, tell me something real
How can we heal?
Children, please tell me why
Why do we all suffer and die?

Children, what is the key to immortality?
What is the key to immortality?
O Children, please let us know
which way to go.

What?
Fruit?
Fruit and air?
Fruit! That's it!
Fruit and air is the key!
Fruit and air is the key to immortality!

Thank you children!
Thank you children of the sun!
Now I understand what I have done!
Now I remember, we used to have fun!
We used to frolic together all day out in the sun!

But now we must go
We are not clean enough to have such fun
We are all sick and suffering
And there is a great deal of work to be done.

Slaughterhouse

Bodies Stacked like paintings
In an art gallery.
One by one cows dangle by a leg.
Man in overalls grins
exposing a tooth
as he clubs a decrepit one with a 2x4
over the head,
repeatedly.

Mid-section wound for blood draining.
A piercing shriek thrives
from the place that had been an abdomen.

One Last Time

I look down at her
two amputated legs
Light green mucus oozes
through the thick metal stitches
curbed into her swollen flesh
An elderly man in the T. V.
room slobbers on himself
The smell from a bed pan
My mother laying there
with her white moonface.

Scrapes and scars from countless shots and I. V.s
Uneaten jello on a table beside her.
The everyday sound
of the heart monitor
Beep . . .
Beep . . .

In the hall
A fat orderly pushes
Rosie to bingo
her arms twitching uncontrollably.

My Mother
43 years old.

Armed with my Teenage
Mutant Ninja Turtle backpack
I look into her paper-white face.
With my finger I open her eyelid
To reveal a watery white ball.
I tell my aunt that she is not in there.

little me

is this the face that gorged a thousand chips
and swallowed up the smoke of endless drow,
all plump and brown just like a rotten pear
terrible, but i sure didn't know.

are these the hands that held the dead carcass
the philly-cheese and t-bone steak done well
that special sauce on my hot wing is what
kept my stank body in such hell.

are these the eyes that slept with K. F. C.
my nose blew for hours upon end,
bronchitis while slaughtering on the football field
mucus remained my dearest friend.

and these fingers that freaked the black and mild
j. reece hollers, "i got dubs on dat"
another says, "naw bruh dat's my ish"
you'd think we were smokin' on crack.

is this the tongue that guzzled Old E.
chased by Hennessy and Wild Rose
the Eagle Scout plates were what saved me
from cops accosting me on the side of the road.

was this the bod that weighed three-hundred pounds
and waddled like a duck on L. S. D.
in pain all day just running out of time
it's hard to grasp that this was little me.

180 Days

Every time that I have fasted for a few days
I sit on top of Calhoun
observing this dead ol' city,
Cincinnati—the city mucus built
streets I've not known nor
want to know, brown structure,
silver sidings, brassy, baby skyscraper
a little bit northward the Ignored and Neglected
Vine St. hangs out, its appearance
the crowning achievement
of mucus and pus, pigs fly
through with flickering lights
strapped to their backs squealing
to the yellow Barr's Pawn and Loan
to begin beating yet another
black teenager.

I hit play on my mini disc
"If you don't know how your body operates you can be told anything,"
recording quality is good,
We sound real good
I kind of feel like Malcolm when
I promulgate my spoken
word over my band's
driving life force-
"Your body is an air-gas engine that does not run on food"
folks start to exit the concert hall
hurriedly, others fascinated by
this crazy guy with colorful war paint on
hollerin' about the fundamental
cause of all disease and death
stay, jaws smeared on the floor-

Down on the streets I see pus-filled zombies
all shapes and sizes
hurriedly on the move,
radars searching for the
nearest Mickey-D's to buy
pure donkey doo doo
and call it food.

Sad and sickened
I take the elevator and go
down, pondering
and float over the pavement
to Brother Air's house, first
stopping for lemons at the Kroghetto

180 days!
180 days of fasting for Brother Air!
no solid food!
makes my four day fast
look like a joke, but
he's been into the
Mucusless Diet Healing
System for over 20 years,
practitioner of breathaireanism
We discuss Jazz
the death culture
being oppressed
by pus-filled zombies
and the future direction of humanity.

Relief

From the reflection of the moon
on my fasting son's fingernail,
at first soft quartz stuck in the mountain,
then a sea of hornblende and gypsum
I await an answer.

Inside intestines formerly filled
with forests of chaos, no longer choke
the oxygen flow.
Globs of filth mixed with lemon juice are flushed,
enema bag left on the sink, *Coltrane Live
in Japan* still playing.

Relief shines in the smiling
eyes of my son.

Air Ode

Oh, Ode to air, the giver of life
That enables existence for me
As well as pink and purple phalaenopsis
Scarlet oak and birch tree

With every breath my red blood rusts
To perfect blackness

My feet like burnt brass
Eyes burgundy to black
Face illuminating purity

Gravitational bloodstream
Manifests a blackhole
Immortality

Breathairean self-existence

Mauve

      Accord

          Claret

              Silence

                  Pitch-Black

                      Searing Soul

                        Peace

Fruit of a Tree Yielding Seed

To you, this shall be for food

Oceans

Child asks: Where do oceans come from?

Vic answers:

Well, the earth did not always have bodies of salt water.
Once upon a time the earth was one big landmass
The whole world was the same temperature
Think of the earth as living tissue
Hue-mans were the blood corpuscles of earth's tissue
Part of a larger, universal host
You know why they call it Mother Earth, right?
At one time unrefined humans could be grown from the earth.
Today, many fruits and vegetables resemble body parts.

Child: Like cabbage?

Vic: Very good.

A cross section of cabbage looks like a brain
Dark grapes bleed juice similar to our blood
We are the Earth

Before hue-mans began eating
We did not age and dye.
Such hue-mans were supermen and superwomen
They did not eat nor drink, they did not sleep
They could fly if they needed
They could be in multiple places at the same time
They existed for thousands of years without aging
Without dyeing.

Child: What was their purpose?

Vic: To shine. It was all about who could shine the most.
Illumination, radioactivity, black holes

      but, then someone ate something.

Child: Why?

Vic: That's the tragic question. Hue-man's eternal flaw.

It is unclear why, but there was some imperfection
that needed to be eliminated.

Once eating began, the desire to eat more arose.
We then existed on grapes, apples, bananas,
and oranges for thousands of years

Child: Fruitarians?

Vic: Yes.

But over time, eventually fruit began to obstruct the body.
Then hue-mans began to crave starchy fruits
Then vegetables.
As more waste was accumulated in the body,
worse foods were eaten.

Child: why did people start eating dead animal meat?

Vic: By that time hue-mans had degenerated quite a bit.

Now it becomes harder to call these people hue-mans.
It could be said that these meat eaters were becoming underdeveloped
humans
Rapidly descending into the animal world.

> You are what you eat.
> Eat dead animal and become a dead animal
> Eat produce and be productive!

After a while humans started to die.
The death of humans negatively affected Mother Earth
Havoc erupted
Death begets death, and the desire to kill was a direct result of eating
The taste for flesh is the taste for dEATh.

As humans began to die from the affect of eating
The earth began to accumulate salty water.

Child: How come?

Vic: Well, one the waste products of dead humans and animals is salt
water.

How many dead bodies do you think it takes to create and ocean?

Child: A whole lot!

Vic: Yes, it takes a lot of death to create an ocean!

Many of the world's indigenous peoples have myths
about the destruction of the world by water

Native Americans, Australian Aborigines, and Dogons
in African all have flood stories.
Egyptians, Hebrews, Christians, Muslims have flood stories.

Child: Like Noah and the Ark.

Vic: Yes, but that story is fairly new compared to many others.

What seems to be consistent is a world of human gluttony and great
war.
Great battles were waged between evil giants and humans.
Hindu scriptures speak of this war.
Egyptian and Greek myth reference such an event.
Constipated Supermen challenging the lives of a
devolved, yet a bit more virtuous, class of smaller humans.
The group of humans prevailed and did away with the evil giants

Child: like Jack and the Beanstalk?

Vic: Yes. Jack and the Beanstalk is but a vestige of these times.

Now, if you can imagine thousands, hundreds of thousands
of humans dyeing at one time, how many millions of gallons of
Salt water would be created?
To people who were used to having a world with no boundaries
It would feel like the earth is being destroyed by water.

A great flood.
A great flood of death.

Child: But, if the oceans are dead people, why do people swim and play
in it?

Vic: Well, we exist in a death culture

In other words, we are part of a reality that revolves around death.
It's hard to call it a culture.
Can you name some death elements of our habitat?

Child: On Halloween people dress up like dead people and scary
monsters.

Vic: Very good! Many of our customs, religions, and holidays revolve
around themes of death.

What would make someone want to dress up like a pale dead thing?
Where are the holidays where children pretend to be immortals and

Fruitarians?
Why does immortality start with undead vampires and goblins?
Why do so many of our movies and TV shows revolve around death?
C.S.I., Murder She Wrote, Law and Order, Homicide: life on the streets,
And what kind of humans develop a genre of movies called "horror"?
Where is the "Immortality" movie genre?

Child: What about science fiction?

Vic: Well, a lot of science fiction focuses on a future of great mucus degeneration

Star Wars has robots, human/machine hybrids, worlds of slimy creatures and aliens.
Where is the world of radioactive, black immortals?
In fact, there are very few black people ever featured in the movies.
Where is the world inhabited by radioactive, black hue-mans? The black world?
But, it is hard to imagine such a reality while eating
Vienna sausages and pork chops.

Child: We should not have started eating.

Vic: I agree. Now we must get ourselves together. But it will take a long time and be a lot of hard work.

But, it's like the song says:

Vic sings:

> *Would you like to swing on a star*
>
> *Carry moonbeams home in a jar*
>
> *And be better off than you are*
>
> *Or would you rather be a pig . . ."*
>
> *(laughter)*

Child: I wanna swing on a star!
Vic: Me too.

I Pledge Allegiance

To the snot
of my slime addiction
And to the degeneration
For which it commands
One mucus
The slimy snot
Indissolvable
With death and destruction for all!

Place your hand on the box of tissues

And raise your right hand
And repeat after me

Do you solemnly swear to tell the MuCus,
the whole MuCus, and nothing but the pUs,
so help you Slime?

A New American Dream

My fellow Americans

The issue that plagues the productivity of America is Deathcare

1933 Roosevelt called for a New Deal

> A house for the family
> A chicken in every pot
> Fresh milk on every table
> Goose and turkey for every Thankskilling Dinner

I come to you today with a New Deal
and a New Dream for America

> Pill bottles in every cupboard
> Colorful elixirs for each ailment
> Pain relief for all children
> Surgery for all Americans
> Superior drugs for every man, woman, and child!

Sickness need not hold back any American from living the Dream.

Yes, we will

> Put a pill bottle in every American hand

Yes, we will

> Provide pain killers for every stroke

Yes, we will

> Supply warm, sanitary beds for every ailing man, woman, and child

This is our moment

This is our time!

> This is our New American Dream!

God bless you and God bless
the United States of Pus and Mucus

What is starvation?

It must be understood
that what we consider
to be starvation is itself
a condition of mucus
constipation.

In a clean body free
from toxic wastes, both
emaciated and obese
conditions would not
occur. In both cases
'starvation' is the result
of oxygen not getting
to the blood due to
obstruction.

Many emaciated people
could be saved if only
they had access to fresh
fruits and vegetables.

The principles of the
mucusless diet must
be understood and
embraced by those
who have resources
to help the oppressed,
and the sick.

Access to fresh fruits
and vegetables
could save the lives
of millions, and the
infrastructure does
exist to provide such
food for all.

263

How many pounds of
perfectly good fresh
fruits and vegetables
are thrown away every
day in U.S. grocery stores?

Such foods are not
given to those in need,
but disposed of in the trash.

The consciousness of
the general populous
and those with leadership
positions must rise
out of the mucus-drenched
dark-ages and walk
into the light
of fruits
and green-leafs.

What would the world
be like without
pus and mucus eating?

Do You Understand Your Immortal Rights?

Put the cheeseburger down
And step away from the French Fries
I repeat, Put the cheeseburger DOWN!

You have the right to stop eating mucus
If you give up this right
Anything you do eat can and will be
Used against you under the law of
The Universe

You have the right to a comfortable transition
Raw and cooked starchless fruits and vegetables
Can be used to aid your body
In this transition

You have the right
To use an enema bag
To aid your body, in your transition.
You have the right to use lemon juice
And distilled water to put in the enema bag

You have the right to Heal Yourself
You do not have to accept
The debilitating, harmful grasp,
of the so-called 'medical establishment'

You have the right to refuse the painful
useless operations recommended to you
by your so-called practitioner

You have the right to be disease free
From the sticky, smelly, nasty, putrid,
MUCUS, that imprisons your body

You have the right to Fast
To stop eating foods for a period of time
To allow your body the time to cleanse itself

You have the right to return to a breathairean existence
The right to ascend out of creaturdom
Into the exalted state of an Immortal Hue-man being

Do you understand your Immortal Rights?

What is this Thing Called Food?

This funny thing called food.
Who can solve this mystery
Why is it making a sick man out of me?

I saw it cooking there
One terrible day
I took a bite
And swallowed it away

So I ask you Mr. Doctor
But I don't mean to be rude
What is this thing called food?

What is this thing called food?
This funny thing called food
Who can solve this mystery
Why is it making a dead man out me?

I saw it simmering there
One tragic day
It took my life
FOOD took it away!

So I ask you Doctor
Although I know you're not in the mood
What is this thing called food?

Grown-Up Pills

The yellow bathroom
counter exploded with
pill bottles, among
them Mee Mee's red
Cedeminafinatrinalin
and Aunt Alice's pink
arthritis pill, among
other words seven-year-
olds can't read. All I had
was my white Seldaine that
tasted like chalk while
leaving a white gooey residue
on my tongue. I always had
trouble swallowing them.

I remember the first time
I tried a grown-up pill,
Mary Poppins sang an
annoying song about
sugar in my ear while
I gagged. As it lay on
my tongue it became
rancid and burned like
a branding iron. Mee Mee
tried immersing a new
one in cottage cheese,
pineapple, and pepper.
Didn't work.

I was so embarrassed tears
poured from my crusty
eyelids and my vocal cords
gave way to whimpers. I
coughed and blew my nose
so loud Chuckles barked.
Here I am at six years
old and I can't even swallow
a grown up pill.

Mee Mee could swallow
five at a time. My Mom
would look like a walrus
wiggling her head to devour
ten. How could I be grown up
if I couldn't even swallow one?

Music (Haiku)

Music is like air
It cannot be seen or touched
It keeps you alive

See?

Squeeze me out
Heat me up
Then shoot me up and let me go to work.

If you could only see what I see,
YEARS of caked on
FILTH!

It's my job to help clean it up.
I'll help loosen this mess
as much as I can.

Uh oh, that's enough, time to shoot back out!

SEE?

That wasn't so bad,
And I may have just saved your life,
For I am the all important lemon enema

R.I.P. Mr. Food Pyramid

Ladies and Gentleman
We are here today to lay to rest
A dear, dear friend
Someone who has been with us
for a long time, for over three decades
Someone who we've depended on
Someone who we loved.

I'm talking, of course, about
Mr. Food Pyramid, Ladies and Gentlemen.

In 1974, Mr. Food Pyramid had made
a wonderful contribution to physiological
enslavement everywhere!

In an age of incivility, turmoil, death, destruction and disease
Mr. Food Pyramid has helped comfort us in our ignorance.

Mr. Food Pyramid told us that it was okay
to eat a piece of chicken
Go ahead and eat that fish
and that hot dog, and that cheese
Go ahead and eat that steak brother!

Would you like fries with that?

He was such a good friend
He made us feel good about ourselves and our diets.

Mr. Food Pyramid with surely be missed.

So today we bury Mr. Food Pyramid
And may he rest in peace

In pieces.

That Mucus

That Mucus
Come on through
Everybody start to loosen
That Super Glue

It's Spira, Professor
not the aggressor
We got to stop living
like the oppressor

Pursue peace, love, and harmony
The *Healing System* is the only key
to a life that is disease free
Shakedown Mucus, and you'll see

That Mucus, That Mucus
That Sticky, Slimy, Mucus
Is the bondage that keeps up down
Today's fashion is hospital gowns

Just frown at the clown as he slices you down
and don't cry until the blood hits the ground

It's like, get that mucus, get it good
everyday, in the hood
Get out the hood and get an enema bag
raise it high like it's your flag

Clean, Clean, Clean, Clean
Get your colon nice and Clean
Very clean!
Mister clean up that fine, French fry cuisine

And then all the girls said:

> *Oh, that mucus boy*
> *he's always talking about health and disease*
> *he told me to give up Micky Deez, and Taco Bell*
> *and I was like—Brutha Please!*
> *I don't think that I could ever stop eating meat!*

Well girl, that's too darn bad
Your story is tragic and sad
Just think about all of the beautiful mucusless times
That we could have had

Don't be sad, don't be mad
That meat eating thing is a very old fad
It's true, ask your great grand dad!

Breathairean Ensemble Intro

The soft gentle sound of Brother Air's wooden marimba

Spira Speaks:

I am Professor Spira and I welcome you into the world of the
Breathairean Ensemble
A world committed to achieving physiological Liberation
While expressing vibrations of discipline, beauty, and cleanliness.

$$V = P - O$$

Vitality = Power – Obstruction

What does this mean?

$V = P - O$ is represented through the music of all of the great deceased
musicians
Louis Armstrong, W.C. Handy, Duke Ellington, Dizzy Gillespie, Charlie
Parker, Robert Johnson, Muddy Waters, Jimi Hendrix, John Coltrane,
Miles Davis, J.J. Johnson, Dexter Gordon, Albert Ayler, Rasan Roland
Kirk, and countless others

Their music represents vibrations of immortality.

My question is, if the music can stand the test of time than why can't the
musicians?

Filthiness is what took these musicians from us. But now we know what
creates this filthiness.

Any food that enters the body that is not a fruit or a green-leaf vegetable
creates filthiness.

The physiological revolution is at hand.
It is time for us to stop eating death and start eating life.

The vanguard revolutionaries are those who learn to control what they put into their bodies.

America is the wealthiest country in the world
And we are always burying the healthy but we never bury the healthy

Death has mistakenly become natural
So if everyone is eating and dying, then why don't we stop eating?

I have a dream that one day all the little children of the world will be able to sit at the lunch counter together in perfect harmony looking at menus
to find out that today's special is absolutely nothing at all
Then the joyful voices of perfect human beings will cry out saying

Free at last, free at last, thank God almighty, my body is free at last!

Haneef exclaims:

Hey guys can we play the music now!?

cymbal **crash** . . .

Peace, Love, and Breath!

Bibliography

Carrington, Hereward. 1963. *The Natural Food of Man: Being an Attempt to Prove from Comparative Anatomy, Physiology, Chemistry and Hygiene, That the Original, Best and Natural Diet of Man Is Fruit and Nuts.* Mokelumne Hill, Ca: Health Research, 1963.

Ehret, Arnold. 1922. *The Definite Cure of Chronic Constipation.* Los Angeles: Ehret Literature Pub. Co.

———. 1922. *The Definitive Cure of Chronic Constipation: Also Overcoming Constipation Naturally.* Greenwich, CT: Benedict Lust Publications.

———. 1922. *The Internal Uncleanliness of Man.* Butler, NJ: Lust.

———. 1924. *Prof. Arnold Ehret's Mucusless Diet Healing System.* Los Angeles: Ehret Literature Pub. Co.

———. 1924. *A Scientific Method of Eating Your Way to Health; Ehret's Mucusless Diet Healing System.* Los Angeles: Ehret literature Pub. Co.

———. 1926. *Rational Fasting for Physical, Mental, and Spiritual Rejuvenation.* Los Angeles: Ehret Literature Pub.

———. 1953. *Arnold Ehret's Mucusless-Diet Healing System: A Complete Course for Those Who Desire to Learn How to Control Their Health.* Beaumont, CA: Ehret Literature.

———. 1955. *The Definite Cure of Chronic Constipation Also Overcoming Constipation Naturally: The Internal Uncleanliness of Man.* Beaumont, CA: Ehret Literature Pub. Co.

279

————. 1966. *Physical Fitness thru a Superior Diet, Fasting and Dietetics: Also, A Religious Concept of Physical, Spiritual and Mental Dietetics.* Beaumont, CA: Ehret Literature Pub. Co.

————. 1966. *Roads to Health and Happiness: Building Strength and Bodily Efficiency, Internal Cleanliness, My Road to Health.* Beaumont, CA: Ehret Literature Pub. Co.

————. 1970 [2002]. *Mucusless Diet Healing System: A Scientific Method of Eating Your Way to Health, with Introduction by Benedict Lust.* New York: Benedict Lust Publishers.

————. 1994. *Arnold Ehret's Mucusless Diet Healing System: A Complete Course for Those Who Desire to Learn How to Control Their Health.* Dobbs Ferry, NY: Ehret Literature.

————. 1994. *Physical Fitness thru a Superior Diet, Fasting and Dietetics: Also, A Religious Concept of Physical, Spiritual, and Mental Dietetics.* 8th ed. Beaumont, CA: Ehret Literature.

————. 2001. *The Cause and Cure of Human Illness.* Translated by Dr. Ludwig Max Fischer. Dobbs Ferry, N.Y.: Ehret Literature Pub.

————. 2013. *Prof. Arnold Ehret's Mucusless Diet Healing System: Annotated, Revised, and Edited by Prof. Spira.* Prof. Spira, ed. Columbus, OH: Breathair Publishing.

Ehret, Arnold, and Fred S. Hirsch. 1965. *Rational Fasting for Physical, Mental, and Spiritual Rejuvenation.* Beaumont, CA: Ehret Literature Pub. Co.

————. 1972. *The Definite Cure of Chronic Constipation: The Internal Uncleanliness of Man...the Effect of Laxatives...the Real Cause of Constipation...Nourishing and Curing "Laxatives"...Conclusion.* Beaumont, CA: Ehret Literature Pub. Co.

————. 1975. *The Definite Cure of Chronic Constipation, Also, Overcoming Constipation Naturally.* Beaumont, CA: Ehret Literature Pub.

Garfinkel, Alan. 1981. *Forms of Explanation: Rethinking the Questions in Social Theory.* New Haven: Yale.

Heinberg, Richard. 1989. *Memories and Visions of Paradise: Exploring the Universal Myth of a Lost Golden Age.* Los Angeles: J. P. Tarcher.

Hensel, Julius, and Charles A. Schindler. 1967. *Life: Its Foundation and the Means for Its Preservation; A Physical Explanation for the Practical Application of Agriculture, Forestry, Nutrition, the Functions of Life, Health and Disease and General Welfare*. Hergiswil, CH: C. Schindler.

Hirsch, Fred. 1994. "Introduction." In *Arnold Ehret's Mucusless Diet Healing System: A Complete Course for Those Who Desire to Learn How to Control Their Health*, 9-12. Dobbs Ferry, NY: Ehret Literature.

Hotema, Hilton. 1962. *Man's Higher Consciousness*. Mokelumne Hill, CA: Health Research, 1962.

Jensen, Bernard, and Sylvia Bell. 1981. *Tissue Cleansing Through Bowel Management: From the Simple to the Ultimate*. Escondido, CA: B. Jensen.

Kennedy, Gordon. 1998. "Arnold Ehret." In *Children of the Sun: A Pictorial Anthology, from Germany to California; 1883-1949*, 144-153. Ojai, CA: Nivaria Press. (Also see Kennedy's article, "Hippie Roots & The Perennial Subculture.")

Kennedy, Gordon, and Kody Ryan. May 13, 2003. "Hippie Roots & the Perennial Subculture." *Hippy.com*, May 13. View it at www.bit.ly/hippie-roots.

Kerr, D. MD, and Ms. J. McConnell. 1991. *Living with PKU*. Inherited Metabolic Diseases Clinic, University of Colorado Health Sciences Center, Denver, Colorado. Accessed November 8, 2008. http://www.medhelp.org /lib/pku.htm.

Klaus, Sidney. 2006. "A History of the Science of Pigmentation." Blackwell Publishing.com. Accessed February 8. www.bit.ly/pigmentation-history.

Kuhn, Thomas Samuel. 1962. *The Structure of Scientific Revolutions*. Chicago: University of Chicago Press.

Lide, David R. 2008. *CRC Handbook of Chemistry and Physics: A Ready-Reference Book of Chemical and Physical data*. Boca Raton [etc.]: CRC Press.

Lowenberg, Miriam E., E. Neige Todnunter, Eva D. Wilson, and Moira C. Feeney. 1974. *Food and Man*, 2nd ed. New York: John Wiley & Sons.

Morse, Robert. 2004. *The Detox Miracle Sourcebook: Raw Foods and Herbs for Complete Cellular Regeneration*. Prescott, AZ: Hohm Press.

Powell, Thomas. 1909. *Fundamentals and Requirements of Health and Disease*. Los Angeles: Powell Publishing.

Ramacharaka. 1905. *Science of Breath; A Complete Manual of the Oriental Breathing Philosophy of Physical, Mental, Psychic and Spiritual Development*. Chicago: Yogi Publication Society.

Warmington, Eric and Philip G. Rouse, eds. 1984. *Great Dialogues of Plato*. Book II. Translated by W. H. D. Rouse. New York: Mentor.

Yogananda. 1971. *Autobiography of a Yogi*. Los Angeles: Self-Realization Fellowship.

Glossary

acidosis: A condition in which there is too much acid in the body fluids. Such acid may be derived from uneliminated pus- and mucus-forming foods.

additive principle: Term coined by Brother Air that refers to the belief that the human organism needs to consume, accumulate, and use various forms of material matter to exist. Modern theories of nutrition and metabolism emerge from an additive concept, whereby it is believed that the human body must take in and metabolize various elements not obtained through the breathing processes to live. Ehret rejects the foundation of the additive principle and proposes his "formula to life" (Vitality = Power - Obstruction), which asserts that human life exists as a result of the non-accumulation and elimination of unnecessary matter. Mucusless fruits are identified to be the greatest eliminators of human waste, followed by mucusless vegetables. Therefore, a mucus-free fruit and vegetable diet will ultimately result in the elimination unnecessary physical obstructions and cellular regeneration.

air-gas engine: Arnold Ehret identifies the human body to be an air-gas engine that is fundamentally powered through the process of breathing. Mucus- and pus-forming foods leave behind harmful residues in the body that create obstruction. When the human organism becomes too filled with obstructions and is unable to get oxygen to the blood, the body comes to a standstill. Thus, mucusless foods are identified to be the ones best fit for humans, as they leave behind the least amount of obstruction and aid the elimination of waste from the body.

albumen: Originally used to refer to the "white of an egg," deriving from Latin albumen lit. "whiteness," from albus "white." It is a class of simple, water-soluble proteins that can be coagulated by heat and are found in egg whites, blood serum, milk, and many other animal and plant tissues. Albuminous refers to something consisting of, resembling, or containing albumen. *See also* pus.

Back-to-Nature Renaissance: a social, counter-cultural movement that began in the late 1800s, originally led by German youth. In the wake of the European industrial revolution, young activists rejected urbanization and middle-class social norms. Inspired by works of Nietzsche, Goethe, Hesse, and pagan religions, thousands of German youth endeavored to return to a more natural way of life in tune with natural laws. This caused great advancements in the area of natural healing, as many began to research and experiment with fasting cures and plant-based fruit and vegetables diets as a sustainable way to live. During the early part of the twentieth century, many Germans moved to the United States and settled in southern California. Natural healers and back-to-nature advocates such as Arnold Ehret had a profound influence on American youth and spurred on the countercultural revolution in the United States, as well as the cultivation of naturopathy, the natural-hygienic movement, and the 1960s hippie culture (Kennedy and Ryan "Hippie Roots: The Perennial Subculture" 2004; and *Children of the Sun* 1998.)

black body: An idealized physical body that absorbs all radiation incident on it and reflects none. Such a body may be identified to simultaneously be the greatest emitter and absorber of energy (see Handbook of Chemistry and Physics 89th ed. 2009).

black hole: A region of space-time where gravity prevents anything, including light, from escaping.

bizarro world: Term used to express the backwardness of modern-day society; inspired by a fictional planet in the DC Comics' Superman series where all social and natural laws were opposite from that of earth.

breathairean: Organism whose primary sustenance comes from breathing air.

constipation: An acute or chronic condition in which there is difficulty emptying the bowels due to an accumulation of hard, dry fecal matter. The term may also refer to the degree to which the natural flow of energy and bodily fluids, such as blood and lymph, is hindered by physical obstructions.

284

dark matter: Type of matter hypothesized to account for a large part of the total mass in the universe.

detoxification: Process of cleansing toxic wastes and obstructions from the body. Such obstructions may include mucus, pus, acids, chemicals, parasites, minerals, and metals, along with negative thoughts and emotions.

diet: Kinds of food that a person, animal, or community habitually eats.

disease: *See* illness.

elimination: Removal of physiological wastes and encumbrances. The term is also used by many Ehretists to identify short or extended periods of intensive waste elimination. These Ehretists use the term instead of the word *sick*, as the connotation of the latter is believed to be problematic. In parlance, a practitioner may say, "I'm going through an intense elimination today!" meaning that he or she is presumably eliminating large quantities of waste and experiencing various symptoms of human illness. Instances of elimination usually spur a practitioner to detoxify, fast, or abstain from mucus-forming foods.

enema: Injection of liquid into the rectum through the anus for the purpose of cleansing and evacuating the bowels.

etymology: Area of linguistics that studies the source origins and development of words and morphemes. Methods include the examination of a word's earliest known use, changes in form, and meaning, and its transmission from one language to another.

fall ("the fall"): Intensive physiological elimination—or healing crisis—usually characterized by a failure of the endocrine system coupled with intensive eliminations on the cellular level. People experiencing a fall may be bedridden for a time and be unable to function in public spaces. Many long-term practitioners of the *Mucusless Diet* experience the fall 8 to 12 years into their dietary practice. Given the severe nature of the symptoms, many practitioners have been known to blame the *Mucusless Diet* for the fall and have retreated back to various forms of mucus eating, including flesh and dairy consumption. Some Ehretists view the fall as a kind of "rite of passage," where the practitioner's dedication is rigorously challenged as he or she pays for their physiological debts/karma. *See also* physiological karma.

fast: To abstain from the intake of food and drink. It may also refer to various forms of dietary restriction, which include abstaining from solid foods (juice or liquid fasting), mucus-forming foods (mucusless diet), animal products, and so forth. Fasting may also refer more broadly to abstaining from modern conveniences or unnatural additions, such as a fast from electricity or the use of electronics for a period of time.

forced fast: Concept proliferated by Brother Air, which refers to a period of time where one's own pathological condition forces him or her to *fast*, or abstain from the intake of food and drink. Air identifies sleep and death as being two forms of a *forced fast*. *See also* fast.

fruit (mucusless): Ripened ovary or ovaries of a seed-bearing plant, together with accessory parts containing the seeds, and occurring in a wide variety of forms. Mucusless fruits refer to non-fatty fruits that leave behind no mucus residue.

fruitarian: Organism whose diet consists of only fruits. Drawing upon Ehret's mucusless paradigm, Prof. Spira identifies a fruitarian to be as a person who has consumed mucusless (fat- and starch-free) fruits for an extended period of time.

green leafy vegetable: Various mucusless leafy plants or their leaves and stems that may be eaten as vegetables.

healing: Restoration of wholeness, health, and vitality. Prof. Spira also uses the word to mean the process by which one can slow, pause, or stop the aging and dying process.

healing crisis: Naturopathic term that refers to a period of intensive physical and emotional cleansing or elimination. Common symptoms include the expectoration of various colors of mucus from all orifices, fever, aches and pains, headaches, dizziness/vertigo, mood swings, diarrhea, vomiting, loss of appetite, depression or anxiety, heart palpitations, and localized pain at the area of obstruction. *See also* fall.

illness: A pathological condition whereby a part, organ, or system of an organism ceases to function properly. It is often characterized by an identifiable group of signs or symptoms and the result of various forms of physical constipation due to the accumulation of uneliminated waste.

Jerry Springer Effect: Phrase coined by Prof. Spira to describe adversarial social dynamics that may occur when a practitioner of the *Mucusless Diet* attempts to share details about their lifestyle with large groups of uninformed people. Initial practitioners often feel strongly compelled to share their experiences with friends and family but are met with harsh resentments and emotionally charged arguments. The proposition of the diet often engenders adversarial reactions by those who feel that their own reality is being challenged or judged. Spira advises practitioners to keep this in mind when feeling compelled to share their experiences with others. He recommends that the practitioner avoid situations where he or she may be attacked by large groups of non-practitioners.

mucoid plaque: Term used to describe an accumulation of rubbery, rope-like, white, yellowish, or green gel-like mucus film that covers the walls of the gastrointestinal tract. Such plaque is derived from uneliminated mucus- and pus-forming foods combined with dead tissues/cells that ferment and putrefy in the digestive tract.

mucus: From L. *mucus* which means "slime, mold, snot, etc." Mucus refers to a thick, viscous, slippery discharge that is comprised of dead and exfoliated cells, mucin, inorganic salts, and water. Also refers to the slimy, sticky, viscous substance left behind in the body by mucus-forming foods such as meat, dairy, grains, starches, and fats after ingestion. *See also* mucoid plaque.

mucus-forming: Foods that create or leave behind uneliminated mucus in the human body, especially those containing albumin. Mucus-forming foods include meat, dairy, grains, starches, and fats.

mucus-free: *See* mucusless.

mucus-lean: Refers to the period of dietary transition in the *Mucusless Diet* when mucus-forming foods are used along with mucusless ones. Mucus-lean menus are generally less harmful than standard mucus-forming eating habits of non-practitioners and are an important part of the overall transition and systematic healing methods employed in the *Mucusless Diet Healing System*.

mucusless: Refers to foods that are not mucus-forming foods. Such foods digest without leaving behind a thick, viscous, slimy substance called mucus. These foods include all kinds of fat-free fruits and starchless vegetables.

mucus-type (fat) physiology: The bodily mechanism of the mucus/fat type is, on the average, mechanically more obstructed. The person is often an overeater of starchy foods and can put on weight easily.

myth: A traditional story, especially one concerning the early history of a people or explaining some natural or social phenomenon. Such stories often involve supernatural beings, events, or archaic forms of logic.

287

Natural-Hygienic Movement: name given to the proliferation of healing modalities that sprung from the Back-to-Nature Renaissance in the early twentieth century. Drawing on the works of naturopathic pioneers such as Arnold Ehret, natural healers and philosophers published many works that covered a host of relevant topics, including fasting, fruit diet, plant-based/mucus-free lifestyles, colon therapy, spirituality, sunbathing, living outdoors, science of breath, clothes-free living, drugless healing, and organic farming.

naturopathy: Term coined in 1895 by John Scheel, successfully put into practice by Prof. Arnold Ehret at the turn of the twentieth century, and made famous in the United States by one of Ehret's students named Benedict Lust who founded a school of naturopathy in 1902. Naturopathic Medicine favors a holistic and drugless approach to healing and seeks to find the least invasive measures necessary to relieve symptoms and heal human illness.

paradigm: A worldview underlying the theories and methodology of a particular scientific subject. It may also refer to the systems of thought shared by a particular community of people. Paradigm shift is a concept championed by Thomas Kuhn in his book, *The Structure of Scientific Revolutions* (1962) and refers to a change in the basic assumptions, or paradigms, within the ruling theories of a scientific community. Paradigm shift has come to also be applied to the fundamental shift in worldview, or thinking patterns, of any community or individual person.

physiological karma: Term coined by Prof. Spira that refers to the physical debt that one must pay as a result of having broken natural physiological laws by eating and accumulating mucus in the body, especially the tissues and bloodstream. It points to what each individual must go through to pay reparations for not only the unnatural eating they have done, but the constitutional wastes and bad eating habits passed down to them from their ancestors. In short, the effects of a person's dietary actions that inhibit them from achieving physiological liberation.

physiological liberation: Term coined by Brother Air that refers to a state of physiological excellence and cleanliness, whereby a person becomes immune to human illness. It is the full actualization of the physical potentials of a person when they become free of their addictions to all unnatural forms of stimulation.

physiological types: Arnold Ehret identified two kinds of human physiologies: mucus and lean (uric-acid) types. In particular, these types refer to the way in which a particular body copes with digesting and eliminating mucus- and pus-forming foods. Mucus types are usually more mechanically obstructed and are overeaters of starchy foods. Their bodies tuck the uneliminated waste into the tissue system away from the heart and lungs, and when large amounts of uneliminated mucus are in the body, they become obese. Lean, or uric-acid, types are characterized by having an inordinate amount of toxic waste, acidity, uric acid, and pus in the body and are generally one-sided meat eaters. The overeating of pus and mucus in this type results in the body breaking down the waste into very toxic chemicals that remain unlimited until detoxification.

physiology: Refers to the study and description of natural objects and the normal function of living organisms.

plant-based: Refers to an eating pattern or lifestyle dominated by consuming naturally grown plant foods while excluding the consumption or use of animal products. *See also* vegan.

pus: From late 14c. Latin "*pus*" (related to puter [putrid] "rotten"), from Proto-Indo-European*pu- compared to Sanskrit. *puyati* "rots, stinks," putih "stinking, foul." Pus often refers to a thick white, yellowish, or greenish opaque liquid produced in infected tissue, consisting of dead white blood cells, bacteria, tissue debris, and serum. It also refers to the substance that dead animal flesh is chemically changed into after being consumed or while rotting. Thus, the ingestion of meat products creates pus residue in the body.

rational: Based on or in accordance with what is determined to be reasonable, logical, and sensible. May also refer to a number or quality that is expressible as a ratio of numbers (see Arnold Ehret's *Rational Fasting*).

raw (raw vegan) foods: Practice of consuming uncooked, unprocessed, plant-based, and often organic foods as a large percentage of the diet.

science: From Latin *scientia*, meaning "knowledge," the term refers to a systematic enterprise that builds and organizes knowledge in the form of testable explanations and predictions about the universe. Also may be identified to be the methodical study of the structure and behavior of the physical and natural world through observation and experimentation.

Socratic dialog: Refers to a genre of prose literary works developed in Greece at the turn of the fourth century BC, preserved today in the dialogues of Plato and the Socratic works of Xenophon. Characters discuss moral and philosophical problems, illustrating a version of the Socratic Method. In common parlance, the term Socratic dialog is often used to refer to an interchange between two or more people—one often an expert/master/philosopher—whereby truth may be realized and discovered collectively through the act of asking questions and naturally allowing reasonable answers to follow.

spirit: From mid-13c., first meaning the "animating or vital principle in man and animals, "and the Old French *espirit*, from Latin *spiritus* meaning "soul, courage, vigor, breath," related to *spirare* or *spira* "to breathe."

Standard American Diet (S.A.D.): Refers to a Western pattern diet, also called Western dietary pattern, which is a dietary habit chosen by many people in developed countries and increasingly in developing countries. It is characterized by high intake of red meat, sugary desserts, high-fat foods, processed foods, and refined grains.

system: A set of connected things or interdependent parts coming together to form a complex whole.

transition: Process or a period of change from one state or condition to another.

transition diet: Systematic approach developed by Arnold Ehret to safely evolve one's eating habits away from mucus-forming foods toward a mucusless diet.

transitional-mucus: Mucus-forming foods that may be used during a mucus-lean transition diet.

uric-acid type (lean) physiology: In the uric-acid or lean type, there is more physiological chemical interference within the organism. This condition often occurs in people who are one-sided meat eaters, where the condition produces uric acid, other poisons, and pus.

V = P - O (Vitality = Power - Obstruction): Equation devised by Prof. Arnold Ehret, which he calls the "formula of life." Ehret's proposition is that the human body is a perpetual-motion, air-gas engine that is powered exclusively by oxygen and that the body ceases to function when obstructed with waste. He asserts that mucus-forming foods create obstruction in the human body, and that a diet consisting of starchless/fat-free fruits and green, leafy vegetables is the only food that does not leave behind obstructive residues in the body and will aid the body in the process of natural healing (see Lesson V in the *Mucusless Diet Healing System*).

vegan: Term coined by Donald Watson in 1944 to draw a distinction between a person who abstains from all animal products, including eggs, cheese, fish, etc., from vegetarians who avoid eating meat, but still consume certain animal products.

vegetarian: Refers to people who employ a variety of dietetic modalities, including plant-based foods (fruits, vegetables) and certain mucus-forming foods (starches/grains, fats). Some vegetarians may or may not choose to include dairy products, eggs, and/or fish.

white corpuscle: Arnold Ehret identifies white corpuscles to be uneliminated, dead blood cells. He challenges the notion that white colored cells are living blood cells that serve to protect the body from disease.

###

About the Author

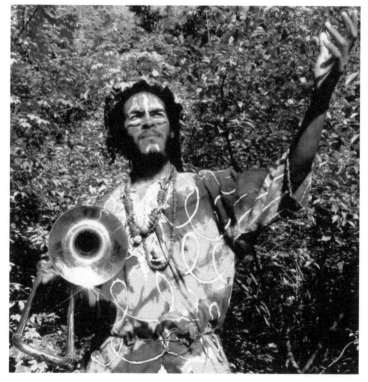

Professor Spira

Professor Spira hails from Springdale, Ohio. He began playing the trombone at the age of 11 and attended Princeton High School where he received the Louis Armstrong Award and earned the rank of Eagle

Scout in the Boy Scouts of America. He holds a Bachelor of Music degree in jazz trombone performance (cum laude) from the University of Cincinnati College-Conservatory of Music, and is the first African American trombonist in the Conservatory's history to earn a Master of Music degree in jazz studies (summa cum laude). In 2006, at the age of 23, he became an adjunct professor of music and African American Studies at Northern Kentucky University, where he taught "Survey of African American Music" and "Music of World Cultures." Spira is currently a PhD candidate in ethnomusicology at the Ohio State University.

Early in Spira's college career, he began to frequent local jazz clubs and bars to "sit-in" and obtain bandstand experience. This is when he first met Brother Air, who, at the time, was traveling to jazz venues and "sitting-in" with his legendary hand-drum rig. In the summer of 2002, Brother Air would have a conversation with Professor Spira and his good friend Daktehu that would forever change the course of their lives. The dialog took place at a jazz club named Chez Nora in Newport, Kentucky during the set break. Spira and Daktehu were munching on the free barbecue when Brother Air started to talk about Arnold Ehret's Mucusless Diet Healing System. Spira was very impressed with Air's claims of eating nothing but fruit for an entire year and ultimately was inspired to read the *Mucusless Diet Healing System* and *Rational Fasting* books. Spira, who at the time was a 280-pound ex-high school football player, was rather ill. He took numerous prescription medications, suffered from chronic allergies, chronic migraine headaches, frequent bouts of bronchitis, arthritis, and sleep apnea, for which he slept with a respirator at night.

One day in September 2002, Spira was in a college practice room with his trombone in hand, looking into a mirror. He explains that a feeling of disgust came over him that he had not ever felt before, and for the first time, he could not believe what he had done to himself. He then vowed to dedicate his life to physiological liberation, and he immediately started transitioning away from pus- and mucus-forming foods. By the spring of 2003, Spira had lost 110 pounds and gone from a size 40 to a size 34 waist. He cured all of his illnesses and was able to quit taking his medications and using the respirator.

In November 2003, Spira and Brother Air met with jazz great and Ehretist Charles Lloyd to discuss the Mucusless Diet. During this conversation, Lloyd insisted they send him some of their music. This pivotal meeting would inspire Brother Air's first 8½-month juice fast as well as the formation of the Breathairean Ensemble. After witnessing Brother Air's fast in 2004, Spira explains that he was physiologically inspired to complete his first 6-month juice fast in July 2005, and his second in July 2006. He concluded his string of longer fasts with a 4-month one in 2007. Though he did not set out to achieve these lengthy fasts so early in his transition, he asserts that the opportunity presented itself and he would have been a fool not to take it. Spira believes that it was the logical conclusion of his submission to the *Mucusless Diet Healing System* that allowed him to pursue his physiological potential.

In 2005, Prof. Spira started to more actively promote the Mucusless Diet and help others learn to transition. Since then, he has become one of the foremost authorities on the *Mucusless Diet Healing System* and the works of Prof. Arnold Ehret (forefather of modern-day plant-based, vegan lifestyles).

In January 2013, Spira released his first eBook entitled *Spira Speaks: Dialogs and Essays on the Mucusless Diet Healing System*. In 2014, he released the first critical and annotated edition of the mucusless diet entitled *Prof. Arnold Ehret's Mucusless Diet Healing System: Annotated, Revised, and Edited by Prof. Spira*. He is currently finishing a mucusless menu and recipe guide, which is projected to be released in Summer 2014.

LIST OF OTHER PUBLICATIONS

Prof. Arnold Ehret's
Mucusless Diet Healing System
Annotated, Revised, and Edited by Prof. Spira

The ORIGINAL Vegan Diet

After almost 100 years, the *Mucusless Diet Healing System* has been revised and annotated for twenty-first century audiences!

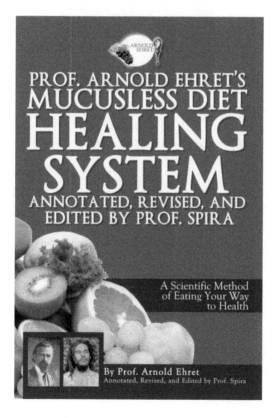

This is a must-read for all
people interested in the Mucusless Diet!

Find it at www.mucusfreelife.com/revised-mucusless-diet

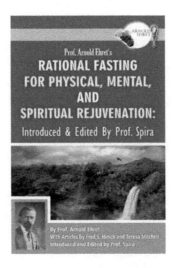

Discover one of Ehret's most vital and influential works, and companion the the Mucusless Diet Healing System. Introducing *Rational Fasting for Physical, Mental, and Spiritual Rejuvenation: Introduced and Edited by Prof. Spira*, now available from Breathair Publishing.

In this masterpiece, Ehret explains how to successfully, safely, and rationally conduct a fast in order to eliminate harmful waste from the body and promote internal healing. Also included are famous essays on Ehret's teachings by Fred Hirsch and long-time devotee Teresa Mitchell.

You will learn:

- The Common Fundamental Cause in the Nature of Diseases
- Complete Instructions for Fasting
- Building a Perfect Body through Fasting
- Important Rules for the Faster
- How Long to Fast
- Why to Fast
- When and How to Fast
- How Teresa Mitchell Transformed Her Life through Fasting
- And Much More!

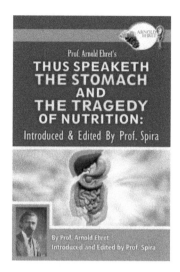 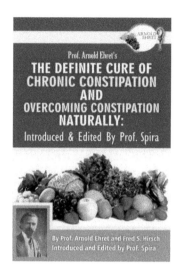

Thus Speaketh the Stomach and A Tragedy of Nutrition

If your intestines could talk, what would they say? What if you could understand health through the perspective of your stomach? In this unprecedented work, Arnold Ehret gives voice to the stomach and reveals the foundation of human illness.

The Definite Cure of Chronic Constipation and Overcoming Constipation Naturally: Introduction by Prof. Spira

In the Definite Cure of Chronic Constipation and Overcoming Constipation Naturally, Prof. Arnold Ehret and his number-one student Fred Hirsch explore generally constipated condition of the human organism.

Visit the MUCUSFREELIFE.COM Amazon store for great
deals on Arnold Ehret's Classic Writings

www.mucusfreelife.com/amazon-store

The Art of Transition: Spira's *Mucusless Diet Healing System* Menu and Recipe Guide

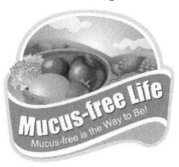

What does a mucusless diet practitioner actually eat? What kind of transitional mucus-forming foods are best? What are the most effective menu combinations to achieve long-lasting success with the mucusless diet? What are the best transitional cooked and raw menus? What foods and combinations should be avoided at all costs? How can you prepare satisfying mucusless and mucus-lean meals for your family?

These questions and much more will be addressed in Prof. Spira's long awaited mucusless diet menu and recipe eBook! Stay tuned!

Introduction

Purpose

Popular Fruits, Vegetables, and Vegan items omitted from this Book

Organic vs. Non-organic

Mucus-lean

Raw vs. Cooked

Satisfying Nut and Dried Fruit Combinations

The Onion Sauté

Filling Steamed and Baked Vegetable Meals

Spira's Special 'Meat-away' Meal

Mucusless

Raw Combination Salads

Raw Dressings

Favorite Mono-Fruit Meals

Favorite Dried Fruits

Favorite Fruit Combinations

Vegetable Juices

Fruit Smoothies and Sauces

Fresh Fruit Juices

Sample Combinations and Weekly Menus

Projected Release: Winter 2015

SPIRA'S MUCUSLESS DIET
COACHING & CONSULTATIONS

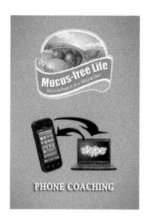

After receiving a consultation with Professor Spira, I was able to take my practice of the Mucusless Diet Healing System to a new level. Speaking face to face with an advanced practitioner was key and a true blessing on my journey. I'm looking forward to following up with another in the future!

-Brian Stern, Certified Bikram Yoga Instructor and Musician

You truly are amazing. You have done nothing but given all you can to help me and I truly appreciate this. Thank you for "feeding me."

-Samantha Claire, Pianist and Educator

"Spira has experienced cleansing on a higher level and passes those experiences to us. He teaches us by EXAMPLE and not only by WORDS, which is rare to find in the world we live in."

-Geargia Barretto, Brazilian Jazz Musician

"When I first contacted Professor Spira for help in practicing the Mucusless Diet, I had many addictions as well as obstructions in my system. I knew it would not be an easy road for me to get started, and I needed help. Professor Spira was able to give me the techniques I needed to start getting out uneliminated feces, black sludge, worms, and mucoid plaquing from my colon and intestines. Within a year I was completely stabilized and elated to be a lifetime practitioner of the mucusless diet healing system. I felt that good! I also had gained the ability to take this system seriously. He then was able to further guide me in dealing with mental and emotional disturbances, social problems and holidays, as well as work and school issues.

His guidance was critical in helping me navigate a world of mucus, pus, and addictions. It has been almost three years now, and I have the vision and ability to practice steadfastly now, and I have much more work to do."

-Tony Bahlibi, Mucusless Diet Practitioner and Educator

Spira has practiced the mucusless diet and studied the natural hygienic/back-to-nature movements for the past 10 years. During that time, he has advised and helped many in the art of transitioning away from mucus-forming foods. For a limited time, talk with Prof. Spira about your individual needs, challenges, and questions. Skype, telephone, or in-person consultations available! For more information, visit:

www.mucusfreelife.com/diet-coaching

WEB LINKS

Websites
mucusfreelife.com
breathairmusic.com

Facebook
Prof. Spira Fan Page: www.facebook.com/ProfessorSpira
Arnold Ehret Fan Page: www.facebook.com/arnoldehret.us
Arnold Ehret Support Group:
www.facebook.com/groups/arnoldehret/

YouTube
Prof. Spira's Breathair-Vision: www.youtube.com/user/professorspira

Twitter
@profspira
@ArnoldEhret1

Visit our Bookstore to Find Books by Arnold Ehret!
www.mucusfreelife.com/storefront/

Spira is now available for mucusless diet consultations and coaching!
www.mucusfreelife.com/diet-coaching

Please Share Your Reviews!

Share your reviews and comments about this book and your experiences with the mucusless diet on Amazon and mucusfreelife.com. Prof. Spira and others would love to hear how the text has helped you.

PEACE, LOVE, AND BREATH!

Lightning Source UK Ltd.
Milton Keynes UK
UKHW011814220519
343147UK00001B/43/P